KU-054-825

Contents at a Glance

BARTON PEVERIL COLLEGE LIBRARY – EASTLEIGH

For renewals, please phone 023 8036 7213

This item must be returned on or before the last date stamped below

8 SEP 2015	10 SEP 2019	
28 SEP 2015	20 APR 2020	
25 JAN 2016		
7 JUL 2016		
27 SEP 2016		
24 APR 2017		
12 SEP 2017		
22 MAR 2018		
- 5 JUL 2018		
07 JAN		

Accession Number

Barton Peveril College Library

320498

Author	Shelf Number
CHOPDAR, & BURTON	378.166 CHO

b   n

FOR
DUMMIES
A Wiley Brand

UKCAT For Dummies®, 2nd Edition

Published by: **John Wiley & Sons, Ltd.,** The Atrium, Southern Gate, Chichester, www.wiley.com

This edition first published 2014

© 2014 John Wiley & Sons, Ltd, Chichester, West Sussex.

Registered office

John Wiley & Sons Ltd, The Atrium, Southern Gate, Chichester, West Sussex, PO19 8SQ, United Kingdom

For details of our global editorial offices, for customer services and for information about how to apply for permission to reuse the copyright material in this book please see our website at www.wiley.com.

For general information on our other products and services, please contact our Customer Care Department within the U.S. at 877-762-2974, outside the U.S. at (001) 317-572-3993, or fax 317-572-4002. For technical support, please visit www.wiley.com/techsupport.

For technical support, please visit www.wiley.com/techsupport.

A catalogue record for this book is available from the British Library.

ISBN 978-1-118-77050-4 (paperback); ISBN 978-1-118-77047-4 (ebk); ISBN 978-1-118-77048-1 (ebk)

Printed in Great Britain by TJ International, Padstow, Cornwall.

10 9 8 7 6 5 4 3 2 1

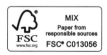

Table of Contents

Introduction

*Y*ou want to be a doctor or a dentist. You clearly love a challenge!

Medicine and dentistry are varied careers with interesting science underpinning daily practice, and with the opportunity to meet a wide cross-section of society and help people through difficult times. The jobs can be tough but they are also highly rewarding if you approach them positively.

Before you head off to medical or dental school, you need to prove to universities that you deserve the chance of training with them. The selection process is long and, to be honest, sometimes unnecessarily frustrating. But if you take things one step at a time, you can get through it successfully.

A key part of this is scoring well in the United Kingdom Clinical Aptitude Test (UKCAT). The UKCAT is a fairly new exam, taken as part of the selection process for many medical and dental courses. It measures your innate talent to cope with the kind of material that you assimilate during your medical or dental training.

Universities want to know that you can interpret written material, perform basic math operations, spot patterns quickly, and use complex information to make challenging decisions. They also want to be sure that you have a sound ethical approach to life. These are all skills that doctors and dentists put into practice every day of their working lives.

For instance, as a doctor or dentist you may have to rapidly extract relevant information from a colleague's clinical letter, calculate the right dose of a drug to administer based on a patient's weight, or interpret a range of lab test results to make a diagnosis and deduce a patient's likely prognosis. And during all of that, you have to behave in an honest, polite and considerate manner.

The UKCAT doesn't expect you to be able to do all those things already but it tries to ensure that you have the ability to learn how to do them when the time comes. Fortunately, as with every test that is theoretically meant to check natural aptitude, your test score improves as you become familiar with the style of questioning.

Practice pays dividends.

We regularly teach prospective applicants to medical and dental school on how to prepare for the UKCAT. Most students are pretty anxious about sitting such a different kind of exam. The UKCAT isn't the sort of test for which you can simply learn a set of facts and expect to do well. Understanding what the UKCAT involves means practising a lot of questions, figuring out *why* certain answers are correct, and then applying that knowledge in the real exam to get your best possible score. We've written this book to give you the framework you need to succeed on the UKCAT.

About This Book

UKCAT For Dummies is for intelligent, motivated individuals who want to rapidly familiarise themselves with the nature of the UKCAT and get plenty of focused practice answering the kinds of questions they're likely to face on the day of the exam.

The book breaks down the different parts of the test into smaller chapters. You can read each chapter in isolation to get up to speed on a section you find tricky, or you can work through the book from cover to cover to get an overview of the entire test.

We also want to leverage our background as psychiatrists to show you some techniques to cope with exam stress. These techniques will help you in the UKCAT and also the other exams you face over the coming years as you study to be a doctor or dentist.

In this book we include the following:

- ✔ Background information on the UKCAT
- ✔ The skills each component of the UKCAT tests
- ✔ A large number of sample questions for each subtest, including the new Subjective Judgement Test, with worked-through answers to help you understand the solutions
- ✔ Complete timed tests to help you optimise your time management, which is crucial in the UKCAT.
- ✔ Strategies for taking tests and managing your anxiety
- ✔ Broader tips and strategies to help you navigate the sometimes confusing world of medical and dental school applications

Within this book, you may note that some Web addresses break across two lines of text. If you're reading this book in print and want to visit one of these Web pages, simply key in the Web address exactly as it's noted in the text, pretending the line break doesn't exist. If you're reading this as an e-book, you've got it easy – just click the Web address to be taken directly to the Web page.

Foolish Assumptions

Anyone who writes a book has to make some assumptions about their readers.

In this book we assume that you intend to sit the UKCAT, with a goal to becoming either a doctor or a dentist. If that's not the case, you can breathe a sigh of relief and put this book down!

We also assume that you're prepared to put in some work. Little in life is handed to you on a plate, and a place in medical or dental school is no exception. If you want that place, you need to have to invest time and effort, not only on this book and the UKCAT but also on the broader application process.

Our focus on the UKCAT in this book means we only have space to briefly mention some of those other application elements. We assume that you will supplement that information with your own wider reading. Fuller descriptions can be found in our sister book, *Get into UK Medical School For Dummies*.

We should mention that the sample questions in this book are designed to help applicants acquire the skills needed to answer a range of potential questions. The questions are not designed to be used by test administrators.

Icons Used in This Book

Throughout this book we use various icons in the margins to flag up important information. Here's what the icons mean:

We use this icon to highlight the most important information and insights in the book. We recommend that you read this material carefully.

Knowledge is important, but strategy can help you answer questions more efficiently. We indicate these strategic shortcuts with this icon.

UKCAT can be tricky at times. We use this icon to flag up potential pitfalls that many candidates encounter. Avoiding these mistakes improves your score relative to your competition, increasing your chances of impressing the universities receiving your scores.

UKCAT is underpinned by a lot of research and testing. You don't really need to know much about it to do well in the test, but sometimes it can be helpful to know why examiners ask the questions that they do. This icon marks out those aspects of the test.

Beyond the Book

In addition to the material in the print or e-book you're reading right now, this product also comes with some access-anywhere goodies on the Web. No matter how hard you study for the UKCAT, you'll likely come across a few questions that leave you clueless. Check out the free Cheat Sheet at www.dummies.com/cheatsheet/ukcatuk for helpful test-taking tips, pointers for how the test is organised, and a few words of advice.

Where to Go from Here

You can read this book from cover to cover for a full overview of the UKCAT. Or you can cherry-pick the parts and chapters that address the bits of the text you're most worried about.

Closer to exam time, you may want to do the practice tests under timed conditions to replicate the feel of the actual exam and check that you're on track – head to Chapters 9, 10, 11 and 12.

The book's structure is flexible enough to be used whichever way meets your needs best.

We also recommend that you do the practice test on the UKCAT website (http://www.ukcat.ac.uk/preparation/practice-test) and the practice tests in this book. Trying the practice test gives you valuable experience with the software that you use on test day itself.

For more advice about applying to medical school in general, have a look at our sister book, *Get into UK Medical School For Dummies*, and the resources on www.medschoolsonline.co.uk. For dental schools try www.dentalschoolscouncil.ac.uk/uk_dental_schools.htm

We wish you the best of luck in the UKCAT and in your future career. And remember: One day we may be under your medical or dental care, so we have every interest in making sure that you do very well indeed!

Part I

Understanding UKCAT

getting started with

Understanding UKCAT

In this part . . .

✓ Decide whether a career in medicine or dentistry is for you.

✓ Understand what the UKCAT is designed to test.

✓ Understand how the test is structured, and get the low-down on the various sub-tests.

✓ Find out how to apply to take the UKCAT.

Chapter 1

The UKCAT and University

In This Chapter

▶ Understanding medicine and dentistry as careers

▶ Getting into medical or dental school

▶ Understanding the role of UKCAT in the application process

You can easily drift into a career without really thinking about whether it's right for you. This chapter explains what medicine and dentistry are like as careers, and what role the United Kingdom Clinical Aptitude Test (UKCAT) plays in the application process for these courses.

Looking at the Lifestyle

Getting into university to study medicine or dentistry is tough. Doctors and dentists are some of the most respected members of society. Medical and dental jobs retain an air of glamour and mystique in the eyes of the general public. And although the reality is often more challenging and more pedestrian than the fantasy of medical dramas, these careers do have some unique benefits.

As a doctor or dentist, you earn extraordinary privileges. As well as receiving an excellent grounding in the sciences, you develop your communication skills, sharpen your deductive skills, and discover all sorts of intimate details about complete strangers along the way.

Medicine and dentistry are two of the few professions where you can incorporate both science and art into your daily working life. A career in medicine or dentistry comes with more job security than most jobs provide, along with an historically comfortable salary.

These jobs have downsides too. Doctors and dentists often cope with the less enjoyable bureaucracy and organisational restructuring. They also face perennial threats to training time, remuneration, and education budgets. More fundamentally, the jobs are often exhausting – physically, mentally and emotionally. Dealing with some of the most troubled and unwell people in the country every day can take its toll. Ask yourself whether that's something you want to do, and why. A bit of honest soul-searching now may save you from agony later on.

If you still want to apply to medical or dental school, you need to overcome one of the toughest university degree application systems. Things weren't always so complicated. When we started out, all we needed was a bit of relevant work experience, solid A-level predictions, and the ability to sound intelligent and vaguely enthusiastic in an interview. If you applied to Oxford, you needed to navigate the little matter of the Oxford Entrance Exam, but if you performed well, you got a two Es offer: as long as you got two Es on your A-levels, you were in!

Barriers to admission are far higher today. To be accepted as one of tomorrow's doctors or dentists, you have to show intelligence and initiative, communication skills and commitment, and resilience and reliability. You need to demonstrate both breadth and depth of work experience, take part in significant extracurricular activities, have excellent AS results and A-level predictions, be prepared to take on large tuition fees with their associated loans, be naturally talented and have practised enough to perform well in the extra exams that universities make you sit, such as the BioMedical Admissions Test (BMAT) and the United Kingdom Clinical Aptitude Test (UKCAT).

This increasing complexity isn't due only to more people applying for courses. The situation is also because universities increasingly struggle to distinguish between good and great candidates on the basis of A-level predictions and results alone. We wait to see whether the recent introduction of the A* grade shifts the balance back to A-level results, but currently many universities consider good UKCAT scores vital. Because university admissions policies tend to change particularly slowly, there may be an organisational inertia against streamlining entrance requirements for fear that doing so would lead to a reduction in the quality of applicants to the best universities. Therefore, UKCAT is likely to remain a key part of the selection procedures for the foreseeable future.

Getting a good UKCAT score is crucial to your chances of success.

We often hear first-hand how worrying the UKCAT is to candidates. The good news is that with preparation, you can improve your eventual performance markedly. In this book we aim to help you do just that.

Applying to Read Medicine or Dentistry

If you've weighed the pros and cons of a career in medicine or dentistry and decided it's what you really want, you need to know exactly how to go about it. The application process is long, and it starts early.

Use this section as a jumping-off point to research the medical fields further. Our focus on the UKCAT in this book means that the information in this section is only introductory to the wider application process. For more detailed information, take a look at our related book, Get into UK Medical School for Dummies (Wiley).

Considering the timeline

In Figure 1-1 we show a rough timeline of when to do what if you want to apply to medical or dental school. Use the timeline to keep the big picture of the application process in mind.

Picking your A-levels

Unless you're reading this book at a remarkably early stage, you've probably already chosen your A-levels. If you still have time to optimise your choices for medicine or dentistry, remember that chemistry is mandatory, and having biology really helps too. Many medical and dental applicants study physics or mathematics at A-level, but these subjects aren't essential for getting into medical or dental school.

An increasing number of candidates sit more than three A-levels. Languages, psychology and business studies are popular options to help potential medical and dental students demonstrate their breadth of ability.

The choice is yours, but you need to expect to score highly in your chosen subject areas if you want even a hope of getting into medical or dental school.

 Having the highest grades is much more important than having many grades. Assuming that you'll do well in chemistry and biology, choose your other A-level(s) based on the subjects you're likely to get As and A*s in, instead of just trying to cram in more sciences. General studies doesn't count towards your A-level total for medicine or dentistry, so you must sit at least three other subjects.

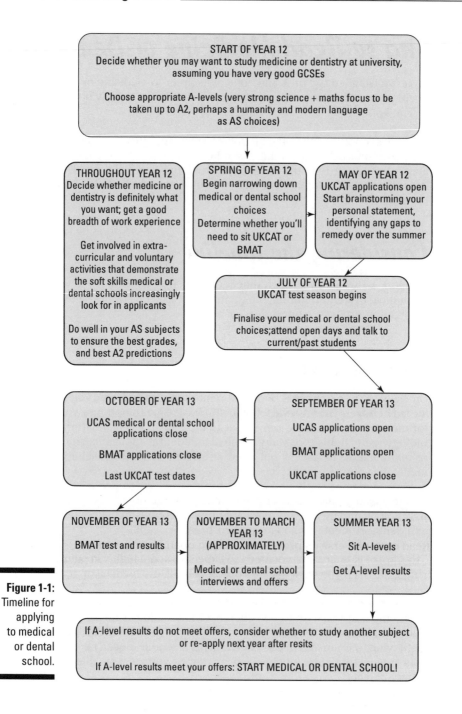

Figure 1-1:
Timeline for applying to medical or dental school.

START OF YEAR 12
Decide whether you may want to study medicine or dentistry at university, assuming you have very good GCSEs

Choose appropriate A-levels (very strong science + maths focus to be taken up to A2, perhaps a humanity and modern language as AS choices)

THROUGHOUT YEAR 12
Decide whether medicine or dentistry is definitely what you want; get a good breadth of work experience

Get involved in extra-curricular and voluntary activities that demonstrate the soft skills medical or dental schools increasingly look for in applicants

Do well in your AS subjects to ensure the best grades, and best A2 predictions

SPRING OF YEAR 12
Begin narrowing down medical or dental school choices
Determine whether you'll need to sit UKCAT or BMAT

MAY OF YEAR 12
UKCAT applications open
Start brainstorming your personal statement, identifying any gaps to remedy over the summer

JULY OF YEAR 12
UKCAT test season begins

Finalise your medical or dental school choices;attend open days and talk to current/past students

OCTOBER OF YEAR 13
UCAS medical or dental school applications close
BMAT applications close
Last UKCAT test dates

SEPTEMBER OF YEAR 13
UCAS applications open
BMAT applications open
UKCAT applications close

NOVEMBER OF YEAR 13
BMAT test and results

NOVEMBER TO MARCH YEAR 13
(APPROXIMATELY)
Medical or dental school interviews and offers

SUMMER YEAR 13
Sit A-levels
Get A-level results

If A-level results do not meet offers, consider whether to study another subject or re-apply next year after resits

If A-level results meet your offers: START MEDICAL OR DENTAL SCHOOL!

Choosing a university

The UK has 35 medical schools and 18 dental schools. Many offer courses for graduate candidates as well as undergraduates. All these schools provide a good standard of education. The exact name of the degree varies a little between institutions, as do the letters you get after your name when you qualify. After completing any of the medical or dental degree courses, however, you're a fully-qualified doctor or dentist entitled to register provisionally with the General Medical Council or General Dental Council, and able to begin working in the UK.

 Choosing between schools on the basis of a given year's statistics on applicant-to-place ratios is dangerous. Prospective students often spend hours searching through data tables that state how many applicants each medical or dental school gets, in an attempt to calculate their chances of success. This strategy is deeply flawed: the raw statistics tell you little about the real nature of the competitive selection process at each university.

The applicant-to-place ratios at Oxford and Cambridge tend to be about half that of, say, Brighton. That doesn't mean Brighton is harder to get into. Other factors interfere, such as only the best candidates daring to apply to Oxbridge and maybe people using Brighton as a reserve option, because the university is based in a vibrant part of the country.

 We recommend that you choose a medical or dental school based largely on its course structure, its teaching style and whether you think that you can meet its typical entrance requirements. The location of the school may also be relevant.

Be realistic but positive when choosing a medical or dental school. You have four slots on your Universities and Colleges Admission Service (UCAS) form to use on medical or dental schools, so you may feel that you can dare to aim high with one of your choices, on the basis that you feel more secure about your chances with your other choices.

 Read each university's prospectus, attend open days so you get a feel for the environment, and talk to current students for an unvarnished report on what life's like for people living and studying there.

If you like the idea of research, consider applying to a school that offers an intercalated BSc degree. These courses often include a strong research element. Courses with intercalated degrees mean that you graduate at the end of your time at the university with a BSc degree as well as your medical or dental degree, at the cost of only one extra year at university.

 Getting a place on a graduate course is even more competitive than getting one on an undergraduate course. Candidates need to demonstrate a real zeal for their chosen career, and many courses expect a high level of proven academic achievement. Researching the different courses to find ones that suit your career to date is crucial to your chances of success.

The peculiar case of the Oxbridge MA

All medical students at Oxford and Cambridge do an intercalated degree.

For historical reasons, the degree awarded by Oxford and Cambridge is a Bachelor of Arts (BA) rather than a Bachelor of Science (BSc). A holder of an Oxbridge BA may upgrade to a Master of Arts (MA) a certain number of years from starting university, on payment of a small fee and without extra study or exams.

The prosaic historical reason for the MA is that it enables Oxbridge graduates to be considered full members of the university, and thus to be able to teach students.

A more whimsical (if untrue) explanation for the award of an MA is that the Oxbridge universities consider their education of such high quality that it takes the extra years for students to fully appreciate its nuances, and by then they are wise enough to receive an MA!

Only in the 19th century did MA degrees begin to be associated with a further level of education.

Perhaps confusingly, Oxford and Cambridge also award more typical MA degrees that reflect extra study.

Writing a good personal statement

The only information a medical or dental school has about you is your UCAS application form entries and your UKCAT and/or BMAT results. You can probably see the importance of doing well in the UKCAT and how crucial your UCAS form is. Most of the UCAS form is fairly straightforward, but the personal statement can distinguish you from everyone else.

Your personal statement must be engaging to read. It should highlight your reasons for choosing medicine or dentistry, how you've demonstrated your commitment to the career, and the soft skills (which we explain in the later section 'Working on your soft skills') you've acquired so far. Don't expect to write your personal statement in an afternoon.

Start writing your personal statement months before the application deadline. Starting early gives you time to identify any gaps and undertake the necessary work to plug the holes, helping you create a more compelling and coherent personal statement.

We recommend you give the statement a linear narrative structure rather than using a bullet point format. Include a beginning, middle and end. Each paragraph should flow smoothly from the previous one, yet also make sense in isolation.

By the conclusion, the reader must be convinced that you have a realistic and enthusiastic view of medicine or dentistry and that you've worked hard to get the real-life experience to formulate that viewpoint. The reader must also feel confident that you have not only the academic skills but also the communication and leadership skills that go along with being a doctor or dentist. Describing the personal insights you've gained by reflecting on your work experience and extracurricular activities can go a long way towards demonstrating an appropriate level of maturity.

Although many universities use a standardised marking scheme to grade your personal statement, good writing skills are still vital: in a well-written personal statement, shortlisters can easily identify and score the areas they're looking for.

Bad spelling, poor grammar and inferior use of language have torpedoed many a personal statement. Bad writing comes across as immature and lacking in confidence. We also suggest that you avoid bizarre or highly controversial opinions, which may expose a poorly thought-through position on a sensitive topic.

Getting work experience

Work experience needs to demonstrate your commitment to medicine or dentistry as a career. In many respects, where you go and for how long you work are less important than being able to explain what you learned.

If possible, try to get experience both in the high-powered side of medicine and dentistry (operating theatres, consultant clinics, cosmetic dentistry, maybe even management meetings) and at the 'coal face' of general practice and hospice and charity work. This not only broadens your understanding of your future career, but also lets you compare and contrast the two settings. If you express these insights clearly and concisely in your personal statement, you'll come across as a much more rounded and mature applicant than those applicants who simply list what they did on their work experience.

Arranging work placements can be tricky. If your school and social circle lack good contacts, a sensible starting point is to make an appointment with your local GP or dentist to talk through your interest in a career in medicine or dentistry.

Work experience rarely organises itself: you have to make the effort to reach out to people and organisations in your local community that can help. Many opportunities exist for motivated individuals. Remember that charities and the non-profit sector are often keen for free and enthusiastic help.

Working on your soft skills

A high level of academic ability and productive work experience make for a strong package. To become a doctor or dentist, however, you also need to prove that you have *soft skills*: leadership potential, communication skills and charisma.

These soft skills improve with practice. For most people, the easiest way to get that practice is to become involved in extracurricular activities that encourage these traits. Think about any sports you do, clubs you belong to and groups such as Scouts and Cadets, and you can probably channel all these settings to give you some soft skills experience. This experience can be a great store of anecdotes for you to recount on your personal statement and in your interview.

Sitting entrance exams such as UKCAT

Almost all applicants to medical and dental school need to sit extra exams in addition to their A-levels. Oxford, Cambridge, Imperial College London and University College London (UCL) request that medical applicants sit BMAT. The vast majority of the other medical schools and nine of the dental schools require you to sit UKCAT.

You have four potential slots on your UCAS form, therefore your choices may span the range of these schools. For medical applicants, that can mean you need to sit both exams. That makes for a hectic and exhausting year.

UKCAT and BMAT test different domains. BMAT focuses more on raw current academic ability, whereas UKCAT assesses aptitude and potential. Performance in both UKCAT and BMAT improve with practice and familiarity, so if you need to sit UKCAT, keep reading this book.

Preparing for interviews

If you've got an interview with a medical or dental school, you're doing well. Most of the cull in applicant numbers takes place before this stage, so you're ahead of most of your competition by the time the school invites you for an interview.

Performing at your best in interviews can be difficult, even if you're experienced. You have to be consistent with the information on your personal statement but still come across as fresh, enthusiastic and personable.

Ask your friends and family to practise interviews with you. If you have a teacher at school willing to conduct mock interviews, that can be a great way to get constructive feedback on your strengths and weaknesses. Dedicated interview skills workshops can provide this feedback and help you focus on the key messages you need to get across to the interviewer.

Chapter 2

Dissecting UKCAT

In This Chapter
▶ Discovering the history and current structure of UKCAT
▶ Understanding when and how to apply for the test
▶ Knowing what to expect on the day of the test

*B*efore sitting the UKCAT, you need to know what's in it and how to apply. This chapter provides that information.

Exploring the Origins of UKCAT

The United Kingdom Clinical Aptitude Test (UKCAT) is, as its name suggests, a test of aptitude, which means that the test is theoretically designed to reward candidates with a natural talent for the tested skills.

The UKCAT universities knew that they had lots of information about their applicants' current academic achievements in the form of GCSE and A-level (or Scottish Higher) results and predictions. But in addition they wanted to assess a wider range of mental abilities identified as useful in medicine and dentistry, including critical thinking, numerical reasoning, and ethical judgement.

The universities hoped that, alongside the existing academic record, an aptitude test would help them choose the most suitable candidates to join their medical and dental courses.

UKCAT is described as a *psychometric test,* which means that the test tries to measure your thought processes or, more accurately, how those thought processes affect your performance in a set of standardised tasks. By grouping those tasks into different subtests, the results show the examiner something about how your ability varies across different dimensions of mental activity.

The UKCAT Consortium

The UKCAT is a relatively new test that started in 2006.

The UKCAT Consortium, a company registered at the University of Nottingham, runs the UKCAT. The consortium's members and directors are drawn from the 26 universities that use UKCAT as part of their selection procedures for medical and dental applicants. This corporate structure ensures that a strong link is maintained between the eventual users of the test results and the compilers of the test.

The test is entirely computerised and physically administered by Pearson VUE, a for-profit subsidiary of the wider media group of Pearson PLC. Pearson VUE administers computerised testing not only for UKCAT but also for a whole array of other organisations and businesses. For example, if you've sat your UK driving theory test, you've already used Pearson VUE's computerised testing services.

A further hope was that the UKCAT would be a fairer way of narrowing down the field of applicants, because an aptitude test minimises the effect of background and schooling on a candidate's achievement.

Sitting the UKCAT

The UKCAT is designed for applicants to medical and dental university courses. The test is a required part of the selection process for the courses and universities listed in Table 2-1.

Table 2-1	Universities and Courses Requiring UKCAT
University	*UCAS Course Code*
University of Aberdeen	A100, A201
Barts and The London School of Medicine and Dentistry	A100, A101, A200
Brighton and Sussex Medical School	A100
Cardiff University	A100, A101, A104, A200, A204
University of Dundee	A100, A104, A200, A204
University of Durham	A100

University	UCAS Course Code
University of East Anglia	A100, A104
University of Edinburgh	A100
University of Exeter	A100
University of Glasgow	A100, A200
Hull York Medical School	A100
Imperial College London Graduate Entry	A101
Keele University	A100, A104
King's College London	A100, A101, A102, A202, A205, A206
University of Leeds	A100
University of Leicester	A100, A101
University of Manchester	A104, A106, A204, A206
University of Newcastle	A100, A101, A206
University of Nottingham	A100, A108
Plymouth University	A100, A206, B750
Queen's University Belfast	A100, A200
University of Sheffield	A100, A104, A200
University of Southampton	A100, A101, A102
University of St Andrews	A100, A990, B900
St George's, University of London	A100, A900
Warwick University Graduate Entry	A101

In Table 2-2, we explain what the UCAS (Universities and Colleges Admissions Service) course codes in Table 2-1 actually mean.

Table 2-2	UCAS Course Codes
UCAS Code	**Course**
A100	Medicine
A101	Medicine (graduate entry four-year programmes everywhere, except King's extended medical degree)
A102	Medicine (widening access six-year programme at Southampton; graduate professional entry four-year programme at King's)

(continued)

Table 2-2 *(continued)*

UCAS Code	Course
A104	Medicine (including initial pre-medical/foundation year)
A108	Medicine (including foundation year; Nottingham only)
A200	Dentistry
A201	Dentistry (graduate entry four-year programmes)
A202	Dentistry (graduate entry, King's only)
A204	Dentistry (including pre-dental/foundation year, except King's, where it is for medical graduates)
A205	Dentistry (King's only)
A206	Dentistry (Newcastle, Manchester and Plymouth), Dentistry (King's; widening participation schools only)
A900	International medicine
A990	North American medical programme (St Andrews only)
B750	Dental hygiene and dental therapy
B900	International foundation for medicine (St Andrews only, one-year programme)

In short, UKCAT is required for undergraduate medical entry everywhere in the UK except Birmingham, Bristol, Cambridge, Imperial, Liverpool, Oxford, Swansea and UCL. However, Imperial and Warwick require UKCAT for their graduate medical courses.

For Cambridge, Imperial, Oxford and UCL medical undergraduate courses, and the Oxford graduate course, you need to sit the BioMedical Admissions Test (BMAT) instead of the UKCAT. (Check out the BMAT website for more information at www.bmat.org.uk.) Swansea's graduate medicine course requires the Graduate Medical School Admissions Test (GAMSAT). If you want to avoid any sort of extra exam, your only options are Birmingham, Bristol and Liverpool.

Does UKCAT work?

It can be debated whether UKCAT actually succeeds in its aim of testing underlying aptitude. Therefore, whether its inclusion in the selection process adds to the fairness of the eventual outcome of determining who is accepted into medical and dental training is also questionable.

In its favour, the test certainly doesn't contain any curriculum or science content. It focuses on exploring the cognitive areas it aims to test. The UKCAT Consortium takes great care to ensure that the test questions are written by appropriate experts, and it then tests the questions extensively for validity and reliability. The UKCAT Consortium also tries to minimise the possibility of cultural bias. We can therefore say that the test has good intentions.

The very existence of the UKCAT does, however, add an extra hurdle to applying to medical or dental school. People from families not historically likely to apply to these medical or dental schools may be put off from applying by the knowledge that they have to sit yet another exam, whereas people from schools or families with experience and knowledge of the system may be more motivated and understand the process better.

In addition, the UKCAT has an entrance fee of £65 or £80 (or £100 for non-EU candidates), depending on when you sit the exam, which may prevent some people from registering. Bursaries to cover the cost are available in some circumstances. (See 'Registering for the UKCAT' later in this chapter for more details.)

More fundamentally, some people question how pure an aptitude test the UKCAT is. A perfect aptitude test should not reward revision or practice. A test designed to reveal underlying mental capability should always give similar results for the same person, no matter how prepared that person is. The UKCAT Consortium takes great pains to emphasise that revision is not required for the test. However, the Consortium's website also states: 'Familiarise yourself with the requirements and question styles in each subtest.' Candidates who reapply tend on average to improve their scores in the second year.

By buying this book, you're already one step ahead in realising that practising any test, even an aptitude test, results in better test scores.

Finding out whether you're exempt from taking the UKCAT

You have to sit the UKCAT if your course and institution are listed in Tables 2-1 and 2-2, and if you live and are educated in one of the following countries: Australia, Austria, Bahrain, Bangladesh, Belgium, Botswana, Brunei, Bulgaria, Cameroon, Canada, China, Cyprus, Czech Republic, Denmark, Egypt, Estonia, Finland, France, Germany, Ghana, Gibraltar, Greece, Hong Kong, Hungary, India, Indonesia, Ireland, Israel, Italy, Japan, Jordan, Kenya, Kuwait, Latvia, Lithuania, Luxembourg, Malaysia, Malta, Mauritius, Netherlands, New Zealand, Nigeria, Norway, Pakistan, Poland, Portugal, Qatar, Republic of Korea, Romania, Saudi Arabia, Singapore, Slovakia, Slovenia, South Africa, Spain, Sri Lanka, Sweden,

Switzerland, Taiwan, Thailand, Uganda, United Arab Emirates, United Kingdom of Great Britain and Northern Ireland, United Republic of Tanzania, and the United States of America.

If your home isn't in the roll call above, you're exempt from the requirement to sit the UKCAT. If you're exempt, you still need to contact UKCAT using a form available on the UKCAT website (www.ukcat.ac.uk). UKCAT will then issue you with a reference number and contact the universities you apply to on your behalf, to let them know that you are exempt.

Getting the dates right

You have to take the UKCAT in the same year as that of your application cycle.

Candidates applying in 2014 for entry in 2015 (or for deferred entry in 2016) sit the UKCAT in 2014. Your test score is valid only for one application cycle. If you reapply the following year, you need to sit the UKCAT again that year.

The logic behind the need to resit an aptitude test from one year to the next somewhat escapes us. As aptitude is an innate talent, it shouldn't vary significantly between years. Nonetheless, the UKCAT rules are clear about resitting, so be sure to stick to them.

The exact dates for UKCAT registration, testing and the publication of results vary from year to year, although usually only by a few days. UKCAT is good at maintaining its own website with the relevant dates for the current year. UKCAT's website is www.ukcat.ac.uk and has a lot of useful information, not just test dates.

In Table 2-3, we show the approximate UKCAT dates within a typical application cycle.

Table 2-3	Example UKCAT Dates for a Typical Cycle
Event	*Date*
Registration opens	1 May
Bursary applications open	1 May
Testing begins	3 July
Registration deadline	21 September
Bursary application deadline	21 September
Exemption application deadline	21 September
Last testing date	5 October
UCAS application deadline	15 October

We recommend that you aim to sit the UKCAT fairly early in the cycle. Then, if you fall ill or for some other reason can't make your initial test date, you still have time to rebook for a later date. An early test date means that you have to start your preparation sooner, but the insurance you gain by having room to manoeuvre is probably worth the trade-off.

If you need to cancel or reschedule your test, log in to Pearson VUE's website (www.pearsonvue.co.uk). Rescheduling is free of charge, provided you give at least a full working day's notice between the time of rescheduling and the original day of your test. If you cancel or try to reschedule with less than a day's notice, you're counted as a no-show and are liable for the full fee (and then have to pay a further fee for the rescheduled test).

Registering for the UKCAT

UKCAT registration is entirely computerised. Go to UKCAT's website at www.ukcat.ac.uk and click the Register Here link at the bottom of the page. Registration is only possible within the approximate period indicated in Table 2-3 (the current dates are shown on the UKCAT website). You will be seamlessly transferred to Pearson VUE's website and guided through a series of online forms to create an account to access the system, register, and pay for the test. Registering is no more intimidating than opening an account with any online shopping site, so don't panic!

The UKCAT application fee is £65 if you sit the test in the summer part of the application cycle, and £80 if you sit the test in the autumn. If you're not from an EU country, the fee rises to £100, regardless of when you sit the test. You can pay securely online with any major credit or debit card. You don't have an offline option, so if you don't have access to one of these cards, you need to look into getting a temporary or prepaid card from your bank or from another organisation like the Post Office.

Many potentially eligible applicants don't realise that UKCAT operates an extensive bursary system that covers many EU candidates for the full test fee. You can apply for a bursary by completing the form at www.ukcat.ac.uk/pages/bursaryApplicationForm.aspx. You can only apply during the registration window indicated in Table 2-3.

Bursaries are available for those in receipt of:

✔ Education Maintenance Allowance (EMA) or 16–19 Bursary

✔ Discretionary Learner Support (or equivalent)

✔ Full Maintenance Grant or Special Support Grant (or equivalent)

✔ Income Support, Job Seeker's Allowance or Employment Support Allowance

When Universal Credit begins, it's likely that its recipients will also be eligible for bursaries, but this is not confirmed yet.

Members of households in receipt of some of the above benefits, or those from the EU in receipt of equivalent benefits, may also be eligible.

Details of any changes to the eligibility criteria can typically be found on UKCAT's website.

To apply for a bursary, you require documentary evidence (generally a letter from the relevant government agency) that you are eligible for the bursary. After you demonstrate eligibility, UKCAT sends you a voucher code to enter into the normal booking system during your application process.

If you've already paid, you may still be able to get a refund. Contact Pearson VUE Customer Services directly on (+44) 0161 855 7409.

If you can demonstrate that you have special educational needs, you can sit the UKCATSEN instead. The UKCATSEN has the same content as the UKCAT, but gives you 25 per cent more time to complete the exam. UKCAT can also accommodate mobility and other needs if you contact the organisation in advance.

Don't register for the UKCATSEN if you don't have special educational needs. Not only is this unethical, but you will be found out. UKCAT does not expect you to provide clinical evidence to verify your eligibility for UKCATSEN, but the universities do require such evidence. Your test results will be declared null and void if you can't provide evidence of special educational needs at this stage. The evidence needed is typically in the form of a certificate from a qualified medical practitioner or another relevant health professional.

Doing the UKCAT

You can find UKCAT test centres across the UK and in the countries where UKCAT is not exempted. You should be able to find one relatively close to you via the UKCAT website.

Make sure that you know where you're going on test day! We can't think of anything worse than turning up to an exam late, or rushing to get there and feeling frazzled, sweaty and confused.

For the UKCAT, we recommend being 15–30 minutes early, because you need to go through some formalities before you start the exam.

Bring photographic proof of identity with you, such as a valid adult passport with your own signature (children's passports aren't accepted) or a photocard driving licence. If you don't have either of these, ask your school or college to provide an appropriately certified form letter.

You don't need to take anything other than proof of identity with you. In fact, you're not permitted to take anything else into the test room itself. Banned items include coats, bags, phones, wallets, watches, keys and sweets.

Although this strict approach seems excessive to casual observers, at least you're now forewarned and won't be surprised when the invigilator insists you leave your priceless family heirloom Rolex in a locker.

For the exam, your workstation consists of a computer, a laminated non-erasable notepad and pen, and a chair. You can ask for a set of headphones or earplugs if the ambient noise is too loud.

UKCAT recently revised its procedures to avoid the need to issue handheld calculators to candidates. Instead, you now have access to a software-based calculator on your workstation computer.

Become accustomed to punching numbers into a screen-based calculator rather than your familiar handheld device, so you don't slow down too much during the numerical portions of the exam.

You can leave the room for invigilator-escorted comfort breaks, but the test is not paused during this time, so try to avoid doing so. The time pressure is already one of the toughest things about the exam: you don't want to make it worse.

After the test, you get your results immediately, because the UKCAT is computer-marked.

UKCAT automatically forwards the results to the universities on your UCAS application that require a UKCAT score. If you want an extra transcript of your results, you can order one for a fee.

You can't retake the test in the same application cycle.

Deconstructing UKCAT

The UKCAT is a computer-administered exam lasting two hours. The test consists of five parts: verbal reasoning, quantitative reasoning, abstract reasoning, decision analysis, and the situational judgement test, which are all covered in Part II of this book.

Each of the five parts of the UKCAT is in a multiple-choice format and is timed separately. This section covers the timings and scoring of the UKCAT.

Timing

Students consistently report that one of the hardest things about the UKCAT is the time pressure rather than the content. We show the timings for the UKCAT and the number of question items in each section in Table 2-4.

Table 2-4	UKCAT Subtests		
Subtest	Time Allowed	Number of Items	Time Per Item
Verbal reasoning	22 minutes	44 items	30 seconds
Quantitative reasoning	23 minutes	36 items	38 seconds
Abstract reasoning	14 minutes	55 items	15 seconds
Decision analysis	34 minutes	28 items	73 seconds
Situational judgement test	27 minutes	71 items	23 seconds

The times per item are rounded to the nearest whole second and should give you a general idea of how to pace yourself through each subtest. Naturally, some questions are harder than others, so you may find yourself spending a little longer on the harder ones. But if you take longer on these items, you have to be brisker with the simpler ones. The UKCAT is designed to allow the very best candidates to complete the entire test, although the pace required to do so is challenging.

If you sit the UKCATSEN, you have an extra 25 per cent of time for each section, but the test content remains unchanged.

Familiarising yourself with the pace required is an essential component of your revision. Try the practice tests at the end of this book under timed exam conditions to see what we mean.

For further practice tests simulating UKCAT's own computer software, see www.ukcat.ac.uk/preparation/practice-test. Doing these tests helps you familiarise yourself with the software environment of the real exam.

Marking

The UKCAT is marked based on the number of correct responses you give in the test. The test doesn't use *negative marking*. That means your score doesn't go down if you give a wrong answer, but instead you just fail to gain on that particular question.

If you don't know the answer, guess! You can't lose marks.

The number of correct responses is scaled into a mark for each of the first four subtests, ranging from 300 to 900. The total score for the first four tests therefore ranges from 1200 to 3600.

The situational judgement test uses a different marking scheme. You get full marks for a question if your response exactly matches the correct answer, but you can still get partial marks if your response is close to the correct answer. This reflects the fact that many situations that test your ethics have more than one partly correct solution. Your final score is given as a band (similar to a grade) rather than a raw total. You also get a written interpretation of the band.

The UKCAT doesn't have a specific pass mark, and different universities have different opinions on what they consider to be a good UKCAT score. (See the section 'Weighing up' below for more on scoring.)

Weighing up

Each university within the UKCAT Consortium can decide for itself the importance of your UKCAT score. Significant variation exists in how the various universities weight your score during their selection processes.

Some universities give the UKCAT score fairly short shrift, while other universities consider the score an absolutely vital part of the selection process and demand high marks. Others expect a baseline level of performance, but they don't award credit for scores that exceed this level.

Universities can also change their minds as to the value of the UKCAT to their overall selection process. For instance, the University of Sheffield required a total score of 2870 in 2011 to be shortlisted for interview, but now suggests that any candidate scoring over 2600 is likely to be considered.

Candidates often worry about this variation between universities, both before they sit the test and after they receive their results. This worry is wasted nervous energy, because even complete knowledge of the weighting formula of your preferred university would change little to your approach to the test.

Instead of worrying, focus on practising as much as you can before the test, and on staying calm and pacing yourself during the test. Then put the results out of your mind. After the test, concentrate on the things you can do to improve your odds through the rest of the selection process, like preparing for the interviews, doing work experience and keeping up to date with any major advances in the medical world.

Think of the application process as the London Marathon and the UKCAT as the equivalent of crossing Tower Bridge. The UKCAT is an important milestone, and you want to be doing well at that stage, but it isn't the end of the race. You can still recover, or fall back, after you sit the UKCAT. After you cross the bridge, put it out of your mind and focus on the rest of the race.

Chapter 3

Taking Tests: UKCAT Strategies that Work

*F*ew people enjoy taking tests. For most people, tests are an annoyance, and some people even find tests terrifying. But if you're serious about being a doctor or a dentist, you need to accept that tests are going to be part of your life for a long time to come.

You've probably already spent a good few years sitting and probably doing well in exams at school. After you do the UKCAT, depending on the course and universities you're applying to, you may also have to sit the BMAT, and then you have your A-levels.

In your preclinical years in medical or dental school, you'll have annual or more frequent exams. During your clinical years, the frequency of testing increases, culminating in your finals. If you reckon that's it, think again: you then need to sit postgraduate specialisation exams to get your Royal College membership, which come in multiple parts taken over a period of years. Dentists too can subspecialise, in which case they must sit further in-depth exams.

Then you have annual appraisals for both medicine and dentistry, with doctors having every five years to demonstrate fitness to practise to revalidate their registration. Most of this work is about continuing professional education rather than formal test-taking, but the idea that you escape tests entirely after you leave medical or dental school is seriously flawed.

If you're reading this book, the UKCAT is probably important to you right now. After all, the test result may be a significant part of whether you get into medical or dental school. Try to remember that, in the long run, if you're successful in your ambitions, the UKCAT is one small test in a long line of other tests. Put the UKCAT in its place and don't let it take over your thoughts.

In this chapter, we suggest some strategies for the UKCAT to help you organise your study time effectively, work out which bits of the test you need to focus on, keep some semblance of a social life, and deal with test day itself.

Organising Yourself

The UKCAT is pretty good practice for life as a junior doctor. When you're on call, you're first in line to be bleeped to do various jobs all over the hospital. You have to figure out quickly which jobs are urgent, which jobs can wait a few minutes, and which jobs can wait until your regular rounds. And while if you're a budding dentist reading this book you'll avoid that scenario, you'll still have to deploy the same time-management and task-scheduling skills in your clinical practice, or face a deeply unhappy waiting room!

Prioritising your time and organising yourself to work within a tight schedule are skills that improve with forethought and practice.

Fitting in your UKCAT preparation requires the same skill. Your life is busy, and you've a lot of things to do. You probably have many things on your mind right now – not only the UKCAT, A-levels and UCAS forms, but also the small matter of finding time to be with your family and friends and, indeed, alone with yourself.

You need to figure out a way to schedule your studying without letting other aspects of your life suffer too much.

Work out how long you've got until your test date. Now think about the other tasks you have to do, and try to give each one the necessary time. Using a calendar, wall planner, or your favourite app on your iPad, map out exactly where you need to be and what you need to do at different times over the coming weeks, including when you plan to be at your desk studying for the UKCAT.

To give UKCAT the time it needs, without letting it take over your entire life, try to set aside some periods to focus specifically on the test. When you're not scheduled to work on the UKCAT, put it out of your mind and don't spend time wondering whether you've done enough work.

'Little and often' is better than trying to cram all your studying into the last few days before your test.

Dealing with Distractions

Be ruthless in eliminating diversions from your study time. We don't suggest you hire a professional assassin to ward off your younger siblings, but you do need to be a bit selfish about your needs.

 Keep these studying tips in mind:

- ✔ Find a calm space to study (home, library, school).
- ✔ Turn off your phone.
- ✔ Avoid social networking websites.
- ✔ Lock your door.
- ✔ Ask people not to disturb you.

Don't give your friends and family the total brush-off though. Explain why you're setting such strict boundaries, and try to schedule time to spend with them. Having some fun with your friends helps you relax and feel happier, and also reassures your friends that you won't forget about them in your new high-flying career.

Focusing on Your Weakest Skills

Most people love doing things that they're familiar with and that they do well. Practising skills that you're good at can provide a sense of mastery and help your self-esteem, but without a clear study plan you may find yourself spending too much time on these areas just to boost your confidence.

You need to score well on all *five* subtests of the UKCAT. A near-maximum score on, say, quantitative reasoning won't be enough to compensate for a dreadful mark in abstract reasoning. (Individual tests are covered in Part II of this book.)

 Spending time on the areas you currently do worst in is the easiest way to increase your total score.

Think about your study time as a resource. You have a set number of productive hours to spend on revision. If you spend those hours working on an area you're already good at, you may improve your performance from 800 to 850, a 6.25 per cent increase.

But if you spend the same number of hours working on an area you're not so good at, you may improve your score from 400 to 600, a 50 per cent increase.

In terms of your total score, you could gain an extra 150 points by spending those precious hours on your weaker areas rather than your strongest areas. Obviously, these numbers aren't guarantees of what score you may get. They're indicative figures used to illustrate the general impact of aggressively targeting the bottlenecks in your knowledge. But the principle is sound.

Practising Taking Tests

The time pressure in UKCAT is severe. One of the best ways to ensure that you complete the UKCAT within the time allocated to each subtest is to practise taking the test under exam conditions. We include two full sample tests in Parts III and IV of this book to help you practise.

UKCAT is a computer-administered test with a software calculator. We suggest that you familiarise yourself with the UKCAT software interface by trying the sample tests on the UKCAT website (www.ukcat.ac.uk).

Staying Healthy

Preparing for tests can be exhausting, especially when you have a lot of other things on your plate. But nothing causes your test performance to suffer more than you being unwell and unable to concentrate.

Here are some 'dos' to keep healthy during your UKCAT preparation:

- Eat regularly and healthily.
- Stay hydrated by drinking plenty of water.
- Get enough sleep.
- Schedule time for fun and relaxing activities.
- Consider using relaxation techniques. Some people enjoy using meditation or yoga to help stay focused. Others may prefer a playlist of relaxing music.

Here are some 'don'ts' to watch out for:

- Drinking too much coffee. Caffeine makes you feel jittery and lose sleep.
- Taking any sort of illicit drug or stimulant.
- Working beyond the time scheduled for preparation. You just exhaust yourself.
- Having too many late nights. Your sleep pattern can become disordered.
- Overhyping the importance of UKCAT. This test is not the only determinant of your application's success.

Arriving for the Test

Make sure you have a reasonably early night the day before your test. On the day of your test, set your alarm to wake you up, even if you normally get up on time naturally.

Try to eat normally, even if you don't feel hungry or you have a few butterflies in your stomach. If you don't have enough to eat, you won't be able to concentrate during the test. Complex carbohydrates are good, because they release their energy slowly across the day. Complex carbohydrates can be found in many breakfast foods like wholemeal bread and cereals, porridge and bananas. The night before the UKCAT, you may want to include brown rice or potatoes in your evening meal. Just before your exam, eat an energy bar or fruit for a more instant energy boost.

Take your proof of identity and some cash to deal with any unexpected emergencies en route to the test centre. Leave home a bit earlier than you need to, in case the traffic is heavy or your train is delayed. If you arrive at the test centre too early, pop into a local café, have something to eat, and take the opportunity to relax a little before your test.

Before any exam, you always see a few people desperately trying to do some last-minute preparation. We suggest that you don't join them, because it will probably just raise your anxiety level. Try to focus on maintaining an even psychological keel. Steady, deep, controlled breathing can help keep you in the zone without tipping over into last-minute panic.

And don't forget to go to the toilet before you start the test, even if you don't think that you need to. Sod's law dictates that if you don't go, you're going to feel the urge ten minutes into your test.

Part II
Examining the Subtests

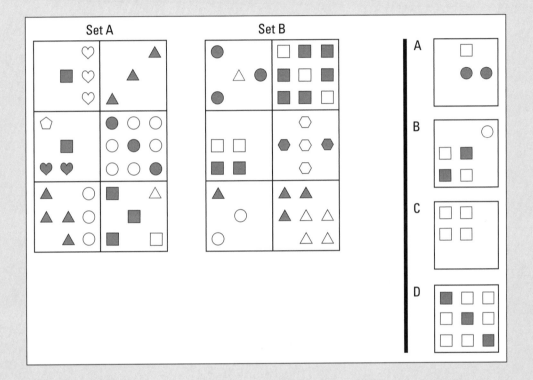

For Dummies can help you get started with a huge range of subjects. Visit www.dummies.com to learn more and do more with *For Dummies*.

In this part . . .

✔ Learn about all the subtests of the UKCAT in turn and in detail.

✔ Get to grips with what the examiners are looking for and the skills you need to develop to answer questions efficiently.

✔ Avoid some of the common pitfalls students encounter.

✔ Work your way through loads of sample questions and check out the fully worked-through answers and explanations.

Chapter 4

Reading Between the Lines: The Verbal Reasoning Subtest

*Y*ou already have the skill of verbal reasoning – in fact, you've been working on it your entire life. Verbal reasoning is the skill with which you understand and work out the meanings of written words, and draw conclusions based on what you read.

In short, verbal reasoning is what helps you understand meaning.

The UKCAT tests your verbal reasoning ability, because this skill is vital for any clinician. Think of the average day of a dentist. She may start off slowly with a coffee, catching up on her email. One message is from a nursing colleague requesting advice about a patient. Another message is from a manager giving feedback from a recent administrative meeting. And then she has a pharmacy bulletin about a newly discovered adverse drug reaction.

Verbal reasoning lets the dentist quickly read all three messages, determine what each person wants and needs, and work out whether she needs to do anything to keep everyone happy. For instance, she may ask a few pertinent questions to get more details before giving the nurse some advice. She may send the manager a quick confirmation that she has read the email and mention a couple of problems that the administrators need to consider. And the information about the adverse drug reaction may prompt her to check that none of her patients on that drug show any early signs of the reaction.

Even before the dentist has left her desk in the morning, she's actively used verbal reasoning in her clinical practice. The UKCAT verbal reasoning subtest tests how well you may perform when faced with similar situations in the future. Universities want to see that you can rapidly take on board written information and use it correctly.

In this chapter, we give you the facts, strategies and practice that you need to score highly in the UKCAT verbal reasoning subtest. We include a detailed explanation of the types of question found in the verbal reasoning subtest, some useful preparation strategies, essential tips for test day and plenty of practice passages, questions, and answers with full worked-through explanations.

Fathoming the Format of the Verbal Reasoning Subtest

The verbal reasoning subtest consists of 11 passages of prose. After each passage come 4 questions referring to the passage – giving a total of 44 questions. You've 22 minutes to complete the subtest.

You have to read each passage, think carefully about the information presented, and use the information to answer each question. There are two types of question:

  ✔ The first type requires you to determine whether each statement is true or false, or whether you can't tell.

  ✔ The second type assesses critical reasoning skills, requiring candidates to make inferences and draw conclusions from information. The question starts with a stem, which might be an incomplete statement or a question, followed by four response options. You pick the best or most suitable response.

The verbal reasoning subtest looks at your powers of comprehension and your ability to logically infer answers based on the information provided – not whether you already know the answers based on outside data. The subtest is about *logic*. This subtle difference is one potential reason why many intelligent and well-read candidates make mistakes in the verbal reasoning subtest.

Determining True, False or Can't Tell

The majority of questions in the verbal reasoning subtest are in the True/False/Can't Tell format:

- ✔ True: A True statement is logically correct based on the information provided in the passage.

- ✔ False: A False statement is incorrect, again based on the information in the passage.

- ✔ Can't tell: If you can't be sure whether a statement is true or false, then you should answer it as 'can't tell'.

'Can't tell' means that you can't be absolutely sure whether the statement is true or false based on the information contained within the passage – not that you find the question too difficult to answer.

Base your answer solely on the information in the passage. Even if you already know something about the topic discussed in the passage, try to forget that extraneous knowledge and answer each statement using only the information provided in the passage. For example, if the text states that London is the capital of France, you need to 'believe' this statement when you use the passage to determine the correct answer.

Working with stems

The stem-type questions can take much longer to answer than the true/false/can't tell questions. This is because you have to check the veracity of four potential answers against the information in the passage, not just the single statement in the first type of question. Fortunately, there are far fewer of this type of question in the UKCAT compared with the first type.

Depending on how your practice goes, you may find that the stem-type questions simply take too long, and prevent you completing the entire subtest within the time limit. If this is true for you, it can be worth skipping all these questions until you've completed the rest of the subtest, but flagging them as you go through for later review. Once you've finished the rest of the verbal reasoning subtest, you can come back and try to complete as many of these questions as possible. This time-management strategy maximises your chances of scoring as highly as possible if you tend to struggle for time in this subtest.

Preparing for Success in the Verbal Reasoning Subtest

A good way to prepare for the verbal reasoning subtest is to practise reading dense, complicated material. Any well-written source of information is fine. The material doesn't have to be about medical or dental matters. In fact, at this stage of your studying, we recommend that you try to read as widely as possible in order to better understand the world around you.

A great starting point is the broadsheet newspapers – in other words, papers that don't have large supplements on TV talent contests or celebrities. Especially useful are the opinion columns of the broadsheets. Broadsheet columnists are paid considerable sums of money to write about topical events and draw parallels and conclusions about them. Most opinion columns are rather biased, because strong opinions help to sell papers, which means that the writers do their best to present a logical argument rather than neutral facts. That structure makes them ideal to analyse in the same way as you would a verbal reasoning passage.

Try reading an article and then summarising the information. Keep shrinking down your summary until you've removed all irrelevant fluff and meaningless words. Half the time you'll find conflicting conclusions, which says more about the confused thinking of some columnists than your verbal reasoning ability.

You need to be able to summarise information quickly, stripping the verbose flesh away from the logical bones of a fat passage of purple prose. If you can do this task quickly, you'll probably find the UKCAT verbal reasoning subtest surprisingly simple.

The ability to rapidly extract information from a wide range of sources helps you formulate opinions for yourself and think widely about the world and its problems. This trait is a useful one for anyone to have, and gives you an unusually lucid and perceptive perspective on life.

Working Efficiently on Test Day

Test day can be unnerving, and you can easily lose concentration and start to panic. Add in the time pressure, and you may end up throwing away opportunities.

Try to follow the tips below to keep yourself focused, improve your accuracy and reduce the chances of spending too long on any one question in the verbal reasoning test:

- ✔ Read the passage quickly but carefully.

- ✔ Avoid skipping sentences or guessing how they finish.

- ✔ Each paragraph of a well-composed passage tends to make an individual point. Try to distil the essential meaning of each paragraph to help simplify the text in your mind.

- ✔ Don't skim-read, because it can force unwarranted assumptions. You unconsciously draw on your external knowledge to mentally fill in the gaps, and ignore what's actually written down.

- ✔ Don't get hung up on things that you know are wrong. The text is designed not to be factually correct but to test your verbal reasoning ability.

- ✔ Don't get angry or irritated with an opinion expressed in the passage. Put your own opinion to one side, stay cool and just answer the questions.

The easiest way to understand how these strategies work is to practise some questions, see how the answers are derived, and discover how easily you make mistakes if you lose concentration.

Practising Verbal Reasoning

In this section, you'll get eleven practice passages, each with four questions, just like in the UKCAT. We include worked-through answers at the end of the chapter. The best way to use this section is to read each passage and then attempt to work out the answers for yourself before reading the answers and explanations – try to avoid looking at the answers until you come up with your own set of answers.

Don't be discouraged if you make mistakes. The whole point of this book is to prepare you for the actual test. Making a few mistakes now means that you're less likely to make the same mistakes on test day.

Avoid rushing through this section. We include full sample tests in Part III for you to do under mock exam conditions. For now, concentrate on understanding the answers and doing the best you can, even if you take a little more time than you will have available in the real test. Speed comes with practice and with confidence in the technique.

The Egyptian with the Evil Eye

(Adapted from *The Last Days of Pompeii* by Edward Bulwer-Lytton)

As Clodius was about to reply, a slow and stately step approached them, and at the sound it made amongst the pebbles, each turned, and each recognised the newcomer.

He saw a man who had scarcely reached his fortieth year, of tall stature, and of a thin but nervous and sinewy frame. His skin, dark and bronzed, betrayed his Eastern origin; and his features had something Greek in their outline (especially in the chin, the lip, and the brow), save that the nose was somewhat raised and aquiline; and the bones, hard and visible, forbade that fleshy and waving contour which on the Grecian physiognomy preserved even in manhood the round and beautiful curves of youth. His eyes, large and black as the deepest night, shone with no varying and uncertain lustre. A deep, thoughtful, and half-melancholy calm seemed unalterably fixed in their majestic and commanding gaze. His step and mien were peculiarly sedate and lofty, and something foreign in the fashion and the sober hues of his sweeping garments added to the impressive effect of his quiet countenance and stately form. Each of the young men, in saluting the newcomer, made mechanically, and with care to conceal it from him, a slight gesture or sign with their fingers; for Arbaces, the Egyptian, was supposed to possess the fatal gift of the evil eye.

1. Clodius judged that Arbaces seemed calm and thoughtful.

A. True

B. False

C. Can't tell

2. Clodius had been waiting for Arbaces.

A. True

B. False

C. Can't tell

3. Arbaces' aquiline nose was typically Greek in physiognomy.

A. True

B. False

C. Can't tell

4. Arbaces possessed the gift of the evil eye.

A. True

B. False

C. Can't tell

Creative Thinking and Schizophrenia

(Adapted from *The Meaning of Madness* by Neel Burton)

At Vanderbilt University, Folley and Park conducted two experiments to compare the creative thinking processes of schizophrenia sufferers, 'schizotypes' (people with traits of schizophrenia) and normal control subjects.

In the first experiment, subjects were asked to make up new functions for household objects. While the schizophrenia sufferers and normal control subjects performed similarly to one another, the schizotypes performed better than either.

In the second experiment, subjects were once again asked to make up new functions for household objects as well as to perform a basic control task while the activity in the prefrontal lobes was monitored by a brain scanning technique called near-infrared optical spectroscopy. While all three groups used both brain hemispheres for creative tasks, the right hemispheres of schizotypes showed hugely increased activation compared to the schizophrenia sufferers and normal controls.

For Folley and Park, these results support their idea that increased use of the right hemisphere and thus increased communication between the brain hemispheres may be related to enhanced creativity in psychosis-prone populations.

5. Folley and Park initially assumed that normal controls would perform best in their experiments.

   A. True
   B. False
   C. Can't tell

6. The results of the first experiment were statistically significant.

   A. True
   B. False
   C. Can't tell

7. In the second experiment, the right hemispheres of people with schizophrenia showed increased activation compared with activation of the right hemispheres of normal controls.

   A. True
   B. False
   C. Can't tell

8. The experiments do not demonstrate that increased communication between the brain hemispheres is related to enhanced creativity in psychosis-prone populations.

   A. True
   B. False
   C. Can't tell

Personality Disorders: Too Much of a Good Thing?

(Adapted from *The Meaning of Madness* by Neel Burton)

While personality disorders can lead to distress and impairment, they can also enable a person to achieve very highly within certain fields. In 2005, BJ Board and KF Fritzon at the University of Surrey found that high-level British executives were more likely to have one of three personality disorders compared to criminal psychiatric patients at the high security Broadmoor Hospital. These disorders were histrionic personality disorder, narcissistic personality disorder, and anankastic personality disorder.

It is certainly possible to envisage that people could benefit from certain strongly ingrained and potentially maladaptive personality traits. For example, people with histrionic personality disorder may be adept at charming and manipulating others and therefore at building and exercising business relationships. People with narcissistic personality disorder may be highly ambitious, confident, and self-focused and able to exploit people and situations to their best advantage. People with anankastic personality disorder may get quite far up the corporate ladder simply by being so devoted to work and productivity.

This suggests that a personality disorder might be seen as 'too much of a good thing' or 'a good thing out of control'. In their study, Board and Fritzon described the executives with a personality disorder as 'successful psychopaths' and the criminals as 'unsuccessful psychopaths', and it may be that creative visionaries and disturbed psychopaths have more in common than first meets the eye. As the American psychologist and philosopher William James put it, 'When a superior intellect and a psychopathic temperament coalesce . . . in the same individual, we have the best possible condition for the kind of effective genius that gets into the biographical dictionaries.'

9. In 2005, Board and Fritzon found that high-level British executives are more likely to have a personality disorder than criminal psychiatric patients at the high-security Broadmoor Hospital.

   A. True

   B. False

   C. Can't tell

10. People can benefit from having certain strongly ingrained and potentially maladaptive personality traits.

    A. True

    B. False

    C. Can't tell

11. All ingrained and potentially maladaptive personality traits can be beneficial.

    A. True

    B. False

    C. Can't tell

12. The author suggests that whether a person with a personality disorder becomes a 'successful psychopath' or an 'unsuccessful psychopath' is a function of his or her level of intelligence.

    A. True

    B. False

    C. Can't tell

Alsatian Wines

(Adapted from *The Concise Guide to Wine and Blind Tasting* by Neel Burton and James Flewellen)

The seven major varietals of Alsace are Riesling, Gewürztraminer, Pinot Gris (formerly 'Tokay'), Pinot Blanc, Pinot Noir (the only black grape), Sylvaner, and Muscat. Over the years, there has been a trend to replace plantings of Sylvaner (once the most common varietal) with Pinot Gris, Pinot Noir, and Riesling.

In terms of wine styles, almost all the wines are white, except those made from Pinot Noir, which are light red or rosé.

A good quality sparkling wine, Crémant d'Alsace, is also made after the méthode champenoise, and accounts for about a fifth of the region's total production. Grapes for Crémant d'Alsace are picked at the beginning of the harvest season, and permitted varietals include Pinot Blanc (aka Klevner), Pinot Gris, Pinot Noir, Riesling, and Chardonnay.

Finally, there are late harvest wines, which may be classified as either vendange tardive ('Late Harvest', similar to Auslese in Germany) or sélection de grains nobles ('selection of noble berries', similar to Beerenauslese in Germany and made from botrytised grapes). Only the four so-called 'noble' varietals, namely, Riesling, Gewürztraminer, Pinot Gris, and Muscat, are permitted for late harvest wines, whether vendange tardive or sélection de grains nobles. Late harvest wines account for a very small fraction of total production, even in vintages that are favourable to late ripening and the development of noble rot. Vin de paille and eiswein are riper still, but made in even smaller quantities.

13. Which of the following can be reliably inferred?

   A. Plantings of Pinot Gris, Pinot Noir and Riesling have overtaken those of Sylvaner.
   B. Crémant d'Alsace is a blend of five varietals.
   C. Late-harvest wines are all white wines.
   D. White wines can be made from Pinot Noir.

14. From the information in the passage, which of the following is true?

   A. There are seven grape varieties in Alsace.
   B. Crémant d'Alsace accounts for a quarter of the region's production
   C. Sylvaner is a permitted varietal for Crémant d'Alsace.
   D. Less vin de paille is produced than vendange tardive.

15. From the information in the passage, which of the following is least likely?

   A. Grapes for Crémant d'Alsace have to be very ripe.
   B. Late-harvest wines are relatively expensive.
   C. Vin de paille and eiswein are also late-harvest wines.
   D. Sylvaner is an inferior grape to Riesling.

16. From the information in the passage, late-harvest wines are never:

   A. Botrytised.
   B. Made from Pinot Noir.
   C. A blend of several varietals.
   D. Single varietal wines.

Nenikekamen!

(Adapted from *Plato's Shadow* by Neel Burton)

In 490 BC, the Persian army landed at Marathon with the intention of invading Athens and mainland Greece. A runner called Pheidippides ran the 240km from Athens to Sparta to summon help, but the Spartans refused to budge. The Persians set camp at the bay of Marathon with a large marsh behind them for defence, and detached a contingent by ship to Athens. The Athenians needed not only to defeat the Persians at Marathon but also to rush back to Athens to defend their city – an almost impossible task.

As the Persian army advanced, the Athenian general Miltiades ordered his vastly outnumbered troops to converge onto the centre of the Persian infantry, which miraculously began to crumble. Instead of pursuing the fleeing Persians, the Athenians marched back to Athens, arriving just in time to put off an attack on their city.

The Athenians had sent Pheidippides ahead of them to announce their victory at Marathon. Pheidippides ran the 40 km from Marathon to Athens, breathed 'nenikekamen' ('we have won'), and died on the very spot.

17. Pheidippides had never run over a greater distance than that which separates Marathon from Athens.

   A. True
   B. False
   C. Can't tell

18. When Pheidippides arrived in Sparta with news of the Persian landing, the Spartans refused to budge because it was the festival of Carneia, a sacrosanct period of peace to honour the god Apollo. Pheidippides was informed that the Spartan army couldn't march to war until the full moon rose.

   A. True
   B. False
   C. Can't tell

19. At Marathon, the Persians strengthened their position by setting up camp with a large marsh behind them.

   A. True
   B. False
   C. Can't tell

20. Had the Athenians pursued the fleeing Persians, Athens would've been destroyed.

   A. True
   B. False
   C. Can't tell

What is the Supreme Good?

(Adapted from *The Art of Failure* by Neel Burton)

In trying to think about what our purpose or meaning might be, a good place to start is with Aristotle's *Nicomachean Ethics,* which is named for or after Aristotle's son Nicomachus. In the *Nicomachean Ethics,* Aristotle tries to discover 'the supreme good for man', that is, the best way for man to lead his life and to give it purpose and meaning.

For Aristotle, a thing is best understood by looking at its end, goal, or purpose (*telos*). For example, the goal of a knife is to cut, and it is by grasping this that one best understands what a knife is; the goal of medicine is good health, and it is by grasping this that one best understands what medicine is (or should be).

If one does this for some time, it soon becomes clear that some goals are subordinate to other goals, which are themselves subordinate to yet other goals. For example, a medical student's goal may be to qualify as a doctor, but this goal is subordinate to his goal to heal the sick, which is itself subordinate to his goal to earn a living by doing something useful. This could go on and on, but unless the medical student has a goal that is an end-in-itself, nothing that he does is actually worth doing. What, asks Aristotle, is this goal that is not a means to an end but an end-in-itself? This Supreme Good, says Aristotle, is happiness (*eudaimonia*).

21. According to Aristotle, all things are best understood by looking at their end, goal or purpose (*telos*).

    A. True
    B. False
    C. Can't tell

22. According to Aristotle, the goal of medicine is good health, and the goal of good health is, ultimately, happiness.

    A. True
    B. False
    C. Can't tell

23. The author of the passage implicitly agrees with Aristotle.

    A. True
    B. False
    C. Can't tell

24. For Aristotle, the end ultimately justifies the means.

    A. True
    B. False
    C. Can't tell

The Laws of Solon

Just as the training master elaborates a general rule of diet and exercise that is adapted to the constitutions of the majority, so the lawmaker, who cannot sit at every man's side throughout his life, devises a set of laws that is best suited to the generality of men and circumstances. Solon, the famous Athenian lawmaker, often complained about the laws that he had written, saying that, because they could not take into account the differences of men and actions, the irregular movements of human things, and the changing needs of one and all, they could not enforce what is truly best for individuals and the state. He also regretted their lack of binding force and likened them to the strands of a cobweb 'in that if anything small or trifling falls into them, they hold it fast, but if anything large or powerful falls into them, it breaks through the meshes and escapes'.

25. Which of the following assertions about Solon is supported by the passage?

   A. He spent all his time complaining.

   B. He cared about the good both of individuals and of the state.

   C. He had not given enough thought to his laws.

   D. He was one of the Seven Sages of Greece.

26. Which of the following concerns does Solon not raise?

   A. The laws do not take attenuating circumstances into account.

   B. The laws do not change with the times.

   C. The laws do not apply equally to everyone.

   D. The laws do not reflect the will of the people.

27. What can be inferred from the information in the passage?

   A. Solon regretted having passed his laws.

   B. Solon's laws applied equally to everyone.

   C. Laws are by their nature imperfect.

   D. Laws should sometimes be disregarded.

28. According to the passage, the author most likely agrees that:

   A. Solon was a wise man.

   B. Solon's laws were fatally flawed.

   C. Laws do not need to be interpreted.

   D. Laws do not need to be revised.

Grapes and Lemonade

(Adapted from *The Art of Failure* by Neel Burton)

A person's beliefs, attitudes, and values (henceforth, 'beliefs') are stored in his brain in the form of nerve cell pathways. Over time and with frequent use, these neural pathways become increasingly worn in, such that it becomes increasingly difficult to alter them, and so to alter the beliefs that they correspond to.

If these beliefs are successfully challenged, the person begins to suffer from 'cognitive dissonance', which is the psychological discomfort that results from holding two or more inconsistent or contradictory beliefs at the same time.

To reduce this cognitive dissonance, the person may either (1) adapt his old beliefs, which is difficult, or (2) maintain the status quo by justifying or 'rationalising' his new beliefs, which is not so difficult and therefore more common. The ego defence of rationalisation involves the use of feeble but seemingly plausible arguments either to justify one's beliefs ('sour grapes') or to make them seem not so bad after all ('sweet lemons') . . . Human beings are not rational, but rationalising animals.

29. Cognitive dissonance can be helpful in that it can spur us on to alter our beliefs in the face of increasing evidence.

A. True

B. False

C. Can't tell

30. The ego defence of rationalisation can be used to reduce cognitive dissonance.

A. True

B. False

C. Can't tell

31. An example of 'sweet lemons' is the student who fails her exams and then blames the examiners for being biased.

A. True

B. False

C. Can't tell

32. Several ego-defence mechanisms can serve to reduce cognitive dissonance.

A. True

B. False

C. Can't tell

The Speckled Band

(Adapted from the short story of the same name by Arthur Conan Doyle)

The little which I had yet to learn of the case was told me by Sherlock Holmes as we travelled back next day.

'I had,' said he, 'come to an entirely erroneous conclusion which shows, my dear Watson, how dangerous it always is to reason from insufficient data. The presence of the gypsies, and the use of the word *band,* which was used by the poor girl, no doubt, to explain the appearance which she had caught a hurried glimpse of by the light of her match, were sufficient to put me upon an entirely wrong scent.'

'I can only claim the merit that I instantly reconsidered my position when, however, it became clear to me that whatever danger threatened an occupant of the room could not come either from the window or the door. My attention was speedily drawn, as I have already remarked to you, to this ventilator, and to the bell-rope which hung down to the bed. The discovery that this was a dummy, and that the bed was clamped to the floor, instantly gave rise to the suspicion that the rope was there as a bridge for something passing through the hole and coming to the bed. The idea of a snake instantly occurred to me, and when I coupled it with my knowledge that Dr Grimesby Roylott was furnished with a supply of creatures from India, I felt that I was probably on the right track . . . '

33. Trying to reason from insufficient data is always dangerous.

   A. True

   B. False

   C. Can't tell

34. Holmes deduced that gypsies couldn't be involved, because it was impossible for a dangerous intruder to enter via the window or door.

   A. True

   B. False

   C. Can't tell

35. Dr Grimesby Roylott had travelled to India.

   A. True

   B. False

   C. Can't tell

36. Holmes could have summoned help by pulling the bell-rope to call for servants.

   A. True

   B. False

   C. Can't tell

Success

(Adapted from *The Art of Failure* by Neel Burton)

Nothing illustrates the emptiness of society's conception of 'success' better than Leo Tolstoy's novella of 1886, *The Life of Ivan Ilyich,* which is, among other things, an acerbic attack on the artificiality and limitations of the middle classes.

The novella begins with the death of a judge, Ivan Ilyich, and the gathering of a number of people including other judges, family members and acquaintances to mark his passing. As these people have not yet come to terms with the possibility of their own death, they are unable to understand or empathise with Ivan's. Instead they begin to consider the various advantages of money or promotion that Ivan's passing is likely to mean for them.

The novella then goes back in time 30 years to depict Ivan in his prime. He leads a carefree existence that is 'most simple and ordinary, and therefore most terrible'. He devotes most of his effort to climbing the social ladder and 'doing everything properly'.

After later suffering a stroke and being informed it will be fatal, he considers on his life and finds nothing for comfort except the friendship and sympathy of a peasant boy.

37. It is impossible to be happy by pursuing the conventional definition of success.

    A. True

    B. False

    C. Can't tell

38. Ivan Ilyich suffered a fatal stroke 30 years before the novel begins.

    A. True

    B. False

    C. Can't tell

39. The author suggests that Tolstoy uses his work to criticise aspects of the middle classes.

    A. True

    B. False

    C. Can't tell

40. In modern society, people tend to have mid-life crises of a similar existential nature to Ilyich's deathbed revelations.

    A. True

    B. False

    C. Can't tell

Concerning Liberality and Meanness

(Adapted from *The Prince* by Niccolò Machiavelli)

I say that it would be well to be reputed liberal. Nevertheless, liberality exercised in a way that does not bring you the reputation for it, injures you; for if one exercises it honestly and as it should be exercised, it may not become known, and you will not avoid the reproach of its opposite.

Therefore, anyone wishing to maintain among men the name of liberal is obliged to avoid no attribute of magnificence; so that a prince thus inclined will consume in such acts all his property, and will be compelled in the end, if he wish to maintain the name of liberal, to unduly weigh down his people, and tax them and do everything he can to get money.

This will soon make him odious to his subjects, and becoming poor he will be little valued by anyone; thus, with his liberality, having offended many and rewarded few, he is affected by the very first trouble and imperilled by whatever may be the first danger; recognising this himself, and wishing to draw back from it, he runs at once into the reproach of being miserly.

There is nothing wastes so rapidly as liberality, for even whilst you exercise it you lose the power to do so, and so become either poor or despised, or else, in avoiding poverty, rapacious and hated. And a prince should guard himself, above all things, against being despised and hated; and liberality leads you to both. Therefore, it is wiser to have a reputation for meanness, which brings reproach without hatred, than to be compelled through seeking a reputation for liberality to incur a name for rapacity which begets reproach with hatred.

41. According to the author, liberality, if done as it should be, doesn't necessarily result in a person being known for his liberality.

A. True
B. False
C. Can't tell

42. The author believes that long-term liberality in a prince means that he spends more money than he has, resulting in tax increases on his population so that he can continue his spending.

A. True
B. False
C. Can't tell

43. The conclusion of the passage is that a reputation for miserliness is more damaging to a prince than a reputation for generosity.

A. True
B. False
C. Can't tell

44. The principles outlined in the passage apply to modern democratic governments.

A. True
B. False
C. Can't tell

Answers

1. A: True.

   The author reports that, to Clodius, Arbaces seemed to have a 'deep, thoughtful, and half-melancholy calm'. Although you can't tell whether Arbaces did indeed feel calm and thoughtful, Clodius perceived him to be so.

2. C: Can't tell.

   The passage contains insufficient information to let you decide whether Clodius expected to meet Arbaces at that time.

3. B: False.

   The text is written in a flowery and archaic style, making it hard to extract the relevant information. However, the author says that Arbaces' features ' . . . had something Greek in their outline . . . save that the nose was . . . aquiline'. The 'save' means that the aquiline (eagle-like) aspect of Arbaces' nose wasn't typically Greek. The statement is therefore false.

4. C: Can't tell.

   Although Clodius and his unnamed companion made superstitious hand gestures to ward off the evil eye, and believed that Arbaces possessed the ability to cast that spell, this belief was only their opinion. Statement 4 says that Arbaces possessed the gift of the evil eye, which you can't verify or deny based on the information in the passage. Note the difference between this answer and the answer for Statement 1. Statement 1 asks only about Clodius's belief, which you can verify from the passage, instead of making an absolute statement about Arbaces in the way that Statement 4 does.

5. B: False.

   The last paragraph of the passage states that *for Folley and Park,* the results of the experiments support *their* idea that increased use of the right hemisphere and thus increased communication between the brain hemispheres may be related to *enhanced* creativity in psychosis-prone populations.

   So, they didn't originally assume that normal controls would perform best. They assumed that the psychosis-prone populations would perform better than the controls.

   You don't need to know whether Folley and Park's initial assumption was that schizotypes would outperform schizophrenics or not (and, indeed, you can't logically derive this information from the text). You need to know only that Folley and Park thought normal controls wouldn't have been expected to perform best out of the three groups.

   The statement requires you to separate out the descriptive portions of the passage from those where the author exposes Folley and Park's own position.

Purple prose

This passage is taken from *The Last Days of Pompeii* by Edward Bulwer-Lytton, a 19th-century author. Despite coining the phrases 'the great unwashed' and 'the pen is mightier than the sword', Edward Bulwer-Lytton is best remembered for the novel opening 'It was a dark and stormy night . . .' His memory is honoured by an annual contest for the kind of terrible writing found in the passage.

6. C: Can't tell.

The text states that the schizotypes performed better than the people with schizophrenia and normal control subjects. However, the text doesn't specify how much better, the sample size, or any derived statistics. Statements regarding significance are therefore impossible to verify or disprove.

7. C: Can't tell.

The passage says that the right hemispheres of the schizotypes showed hugely increased activation compared with those of the people with schizophrenia and normal controls. However, the text doesn't specify which of the people with schizophrenia and normal controls showed higher activation.

Although the answer to this question would almost certainly be present in the full results of the experiment, the answer isn't available in the text provided.

8. A: True.

The text says that, even for Folley and Park, the results *support the idea* that increased use of the right hemisphere and thus increased communication between the brain hemispheres may be related to enhanced creativity in psychosis-prone populations.

This question is a reminder to be careful not to over-interpret the passage.

If the experiment's results didn't provide even the experimenters with enough confidence to assert this statement's veracity (the results are merely couched as 'supporting' the idea), then you certainly can't draw such a firm conclusion solely from the information provided in the passage.

You may be tempted to assume that the experiment's results are valid and universal, but because the passage doesn't imply that they are, you can't make this assumption.

9. B: False.

Board and Fritzon found that high-level British executives were more likely to have one of three personality disorders compared with criminal psychiatric patients at the high-security Broadmoor Hospital.

It's logically possible for the criminal population to have higher levels of other personality disorders not reviewed in this study, and therefore to have a higher level of personality disorder overall.

10. A: True.

The text says that although personality disorders can lead to distress and impairment, they can also enable a person to achieve highly within certain fields.

11. C: Can't tell.

You can't conclude this statement from the passage, which is both hypothetical and partial in this regard: 'It is certainly possible to envisage that people could benefit from certain strongly ingrained and potentially maladaptive personality traits.'

12. A: True.

The author quotes William James in saying that: 'When a superior intellect and a psychopathic temperament coalesce . . . in the same individual, we have the best possible condition for the kind of effective genius that gets into the biographical dictionaries.'

13. C: Late-harvest wines are all white wines.

The key here is not to be taken aback by the use of unfamiliar foreign or specialist terms.

The text does say that 'Over the years, there has been a trend to replace plantings of Sylvaner (once the most common varietal) with Pinot Gris, Pinot Noir, and Riesling', but you cannot reliably infer that plantings of Pinot Gris, Pinot Noir and Riesling have overtaken those of Sylvaner. Even though Sylvaner is in decline and is no longer the most common varietal, it could be that plantings of Sylvaner are (still) more important than those of Pinot Gris, Pinot Noir and Riesling combined, so the answer cannot be A.

The text says that permitted varietals for Crémant d'Alsace include Pinot Blanc, Pinot Gris, Pinot Noir, Riesling and Chardonnay, but this need not mean that Crémant d'Alsace is necessarily or even mostly a blend of all five varietals. For example, it could be that most Crémant d'Alsace is 100 per cent Chardonnay, which means B must be incorrect.

The text says that 'almost all the wines are white except those made from Pinot Noir, which are light red or rosé'. Although it may nonetheless be possible to make a white wine from Pinot Noir, you cannot reliably infer this from the text, so you can exclude option D.

What you *can* reliably infer is that late-harvest wines are all white wines, since they can only be made from the four 'noble varietals' and not from Pinot Noir, which is the only varietal from which red and rosé wines are made. Therefore, the correct answer is C.

14. D: Less vin de paille is produced than vendange tardive.

    The text says that, 'Late harvest wines account for a very small fraction of total production, even in vintages that are favourable to late ripening and the development of noble rot.' It then goes on to say that vin de paille and eiswein are also made, but in even smaller quantities.

    According to the text, there are seven *major* varietals in Alsace, not seven varietals in total, so statement A is not the answer. Crémant d'Alsace accounts for one-fifth of production, not one-quarter, excluding option B. The grape varieties permitted for Crémant d'Alsace are Pinot Blanc, Pinot Gris, Pinot Noir, Riesling and Chardonnay, thus making answer C wrong.

15. A: Grapes for Crémant d'Alsace have to be very ripe.

    The text says that grapes for Crémant d'Alsace are picked at the beginning of the harvest season, suggesting that they are not very ripe.

    Because late-harvest wines are made in small quantities (even in favourable vintages), they are likely to be relatively expensive, making B unlikely to be the best answer.

    The text says that 'vin de paille and eiswein are riper still', suggesting that they are also late-harvest wines, which means option C is wrong.

    The text says that, 'Over the years, there has been a trend to replace plantings of Sylvaner (once the most common varietal) with Pinot Gris, Pinot Noir, and Riesling', suggesting that Riesling is in fact a superior grape to Sylvaner, excluding answer D.

16. B: Made from Pinot Noir.

    The text clearly states that, 'Only the four so-called "noble" varietals, namely, Riesling, Gewürztraminer, Pinot Gris, and Muscat, are permitted for late harvest wines'.

    On the other hand, we are told that sélection de grains nobles (a style of late-harvest wine) is made from botrytised grapes, so option A can be ruled out.

    There is nothing in the text to suggest that late-harvest wines are either single-varietal wines or a blend of several varietals, and in actual fact they can be either. The lack of information in the text on these points allows both the C and D answers to be ruled out.

17. B: False.

    In the first paragraph, the text says that when the Persian army landed at Marathon, Pheidippides ran 240 kilometres from Athens to Sparta to summon help. Then in the last paragraph, the text says that the distance from Marathon to Athens is 40 kilometres.

    Because modern marathon races are based on the distance between Marathon and Athens, you may have the understandable misconception that 40 kilometres is the longest distance that Pheidippides had ever completed. However, the passage points out that the run from Marathon to Athens was the second, considerably shorter, leg of a much greater journey.

18. C: Can't tell.

This statement happens to be true, but you can't infer it from the text. Never use your outside knowledge to determine whether a statement is true.

19. A: True.

The text clearly says that the Persians set up camp at the bay of Marathon, with a large marsh behind them for defence, thus strengthening their position.

20. C: Can't tell.

The text does say that, instead of pursuing the fleeing Persians, the Athenians marched back to Athens and arrived just in time to put off an attack on their city.

However, the attack may not have been successful, or the city may not have been destroyed, or fewer men may have been sufficient to put off the attack. Therefore, based solely on the information in the passage, you can't tell whether the statement is true.

21. A: True.

The text states that 'For Aristotle, a thing is best understood by looking at its end, goal, or purpose (*telos*).' As the statement is not otherwise modified or qualified within the passage, you're logically justified in assuming that the statement is an absolute, applying to all things.

22. A: True.

In the second paragraph, the text says that, according to Aristotle, the goal of medicine is good health.

In the third paragraph, the text implies that, according to Aristotle, happiness is, or should be, the ultimate goal of all human activity.

23. A: True.

The author begins by saying that, in trying to think about what our purpose or meaning may be, a good place to start is with Aristotle's *Nicomachean Ethics*.

The author tends to speak for Aristotle.

24. C: Can't tell.

You can't infer this from the text. For example, there may be a higher principle for humans than the supreme good.

25. B: He cared about the good both of individuals and of the state.

This passage is very short compared with some others. However, this does not mean it is easy to understand. The UKCAT can vary the length of a passage, and shorter passages tend to be correspondingly more complex and dense.

The passage states that Solon complained that the laws 'could not enforce what is truly best for individuals and the state'.

Although the passage states that Solon *often* complained about his laws, this does not mean that he spent *all* his time complaining, so option A is not the best answer.

Although Solon often complained about his laws, this need not mean that had not given them enough thought. In fact, the passage suggests quite the opposite, so answer C is incorrect.

Finally, Solon was indeed one of the Seven Sages of Greece, but this is not supported by the passage, making D incorrect. Remember that you should not bring in your outside knowledge to determine whether an answer is right or wrong. Make the determination solely on the logic of the passage itself.

26. D: The laws do not reflect the will of the people.

    According to the passage, Solon complained about the laws because they could not take into account 'the differences of men and actions'. This excludes option A. He also said the laws do not take into account 'the changing needs of one and all', so we can also rule out answer B. He 'regretted their lack of binding force' on powerful people who are able to 'break through the meshes and escape', so answer C is wrong.

    On the other hand, the will of the people is not mentioned anywhere, so answer D is correct.

27. C: Laws are by their nature imperfect.

    Although Solon did complain about his laws, you cannot infer that he regretted having passed them, just as someone might complain about their spouse without regretting having married this person. We can therefore rule out A.

    The last sentence in the passage basically says that powerful people can escape the law, which means that Solon's laws did *not* apply equally to everyone. B is therefore wrong.

    Although the passage may *suggest* that laws should sometimes be disregarded, this cannot be reliably inferred, so we should also rule out D.

    Therefore, the only possible answer is C.

28. A: Solon was a wise man.

    The author states that the lawmaker 'devises a set of laws that is best suited to the generality of men and circumstances' and then immediately goes on to discuss and even to quote Solon, who he introduces as 'the famous Athenian lawmaker'. He portrays Solon as a thoughtful and insightful man.

    Since some of the problems mentioned are that laws do not take attenuating circumstances into account and do not change with the times, it is likely that the author believes that laws *do* need to be interpreted and revised. This means that answers C and D can both be excluded.

There is nothing to suggest that the author thinks that Solon's laws were flawed. The concerns raised were about laws in general, not Solon's laws in particular, so B can also be ruled out.

29. A: True.

    You can infer so much from the text, which states that cognitive dissonance can be reduced by adapting (changing) your old beliefs. This isn't an intuitive leap requiring assumptions or outside information, but a direct and unambiguous logical corollary of the information provided in the passage.

    This example highlights the subtleties of some of the harder questions of the verbal reasoning subtest.

30. A: True.

    The text clearly states that to reduce cognitive dissonance, a person may either adapt her old beliefs or maintain the status quo by justifying or 'rationalising' her new beliefs.

31. B: False.

    This is in fact 'sour grapes', the use of feeble but seemingly plausible arguments to justify new beliefs (in this case, the belief that 'I failed my exams').

32. C: Can't tell.

    Several ego-defence mechanisms can serve to reduce cognitive dissonance, but you can't infer this from the text.

    Note the difference in how this answer is reached compared with answer 29. You can answer question 32 as 'true' only by drawing on outside knowledge, but you can answer question 29 as 'true' based purely on the information in the passage and without any outside knowledge.

33. C: Can't tell.

    This statement is challenging to answer correctly. First, it's a brave reader who goes up against Sherlock Holmes in a battle of logic!

    More confusingly, on a meta-level, you need to determine the truth of a fundamental axiom upon which the entire verbal reasoning subtest is based. That is, you need to use the very principle of the axiom itself to answer whether it is true or not. In fact, the passage contains insufficient data for you to decide whether the universal axiom presented in the statement is true or false. Therefore the answer is 'can't tell'.

    Always separate out your external sources of knowledge from the information provided in the passage, and use only the latter to answer the questions.

34. A: True.

    In the second paragraph, Holmes admits to having initially been on the wrong scent, and tangentially mentions the involvement of gypsies as being part of this mistake. At the start of the third paragraph, Holmes says he reconsidered this belief when he realised that whatever danger threatened the occupant of the room couldn't have entered via the window or door. Putting these two elements together means that Holmes excluded the involvement of gypsies on the basis of it being impossible for a dangerous intruder to enter the room through the window or door.

35. C: Can't tell.

The passage says that Dr Grimesby Roylott had a supply of snakes from India, but makes no comment as to whether he'd personally visited that country.

36. B: False.

The passage states that the bell-rope was a dummy. Therefore, Holmes couldn't have used the rope to summon servants.

37. C: Can't tell.

You can't infer this from the text. We are told that Ivan doesn't find comfort in his conventionally successful life, but we cannot definitively extrapolate this to the entire population. While the opening paragraph describes Ivan's life as an illustration of the emptiness of society's definition of success, this cannot be used to absolutely declare that it is not possible to be happy by aiming to achieve success.

38. B: False.

The story opens at Ivan's funeral and then flashes backs to a time 30 years earlier. We are not told when the stroke took place, only that it was later than the 30-year period. Of course, intuitively, you would surmise that it was very close to the time of his funeral, but you cannot logically be certain of this. However, it being later than the 30-year timeframe is sufficient to prove the statement false.

39. A: True.

The opening paragraph has the author describing one of Tolstoy's novellas as 'an acerbic attack on the artificiality and limitations of the middle classes'.

40. C: Can't tell.

This seems intuitively correct, if you agree with the perspective of the author of the passage, but cannot be conclusively proven from the text.

41. A: True.

The passage is quite dense, with many subordinate clauses, which makes it challenging to read and to extract information from. The first paragraph includes the lengthy sentence, 'Nevertheless, liberality exercised in a way that does not bring you the reputation for it, injures you; for if one exercises it honestly and as it should be exercised, it may not become known, and you will not avoid the reproach of its opposite.'

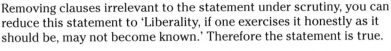

Removing clauses irrelevant to the statement under scrutiny, you can reduce this statement to 'Liberality, if one exercises it honestly as it should be, may not become known.' Therefore the statement is true.

Although you don't need to understand the term 'liberality' to answer the question, you may want to understand that the term, as used in the context in the passage, refers to spending money in large quantities on many different projects, from public buildings and works, to charity, to having a large staff.

42. A: True.

The relevant information is in the second paragraph: 'anyone wishing to maintain among men the name of liberal is obliged to avoid no attribute of magnificence; so that a prince thus inclined will consume in such acts all his property, and will be compelled in the end, if he wish to maintain the name of liberal, to unduly weigh down his people, and tax them, and do everything he can to get money'.

You can simplify this information logically to 'Anyone trying to maintain a liberal reputation is inclined to consume all his property, and to tax his people to get money.' You can now see easily that the statement is true.

43. B: False.

The passage concludes the opposite. The passage suggests that because of the need to have onerous tax rises to maintain high levels of expenditure, liberality eventually results in people hating the prince and considering him wrong. Being miserly also results in people considering the prince wrong, but because tax rises have been avoided the people don't hate the prince as well.

Therefore being liberal causes more damage to the prince's reputation than being miserly.

44. C: Can't tell.

The passage, unsurprisingly for one written during the Italian Renaissance, draws no parallels with modern democratic government. Although you can theorise that the same basic principles of wise economic management apply to the popularity of an elected government as much as they did to Florentine nobility, you can't state this for certain based solely on the information provided in the passage.

Princely behaviour

Niccolò Machiavelli wrote *The Prince* during the early part of the 16th century. Machiavelli dedicated the text to a member of the ruling Florentine Medici family. To the family's detractors, the behaviour of the Medici became a byword for ruthlessness and corruption. To their advocates, the Medici were successful rulers who expanded the power of the states they governed and sponsored much of the cultural efflorescence of the Italian Renaissance.

Machiavelli's work tends to split observers in a similar way. Some view his writing as a triumph of realism and practicality over grandiose ambition, and thus a model for prudent government. Others dislike the cynicism underlying much of the work and the lack of a consistent ethical direction to its advice.

The Prince is still a popular work and highlights many of the tensions inherent in any governing system, including democracies.

Chapter 5

Making Things Add Up: The Quantitative Reasoning Subtest

*I*f you plan to apply for medical or dental school, you've almost certainly already got a good GCSE in maths. The quantitative reasoning subtest in the UKCAT doesn't draw on any skills beyond GCSE maths, so with a bit of practice you should do really well in this test.

At first glance you may think that the ability to comfortably manipulate numbers has little to do with medicine or dentistry, but maths crops up in all sorts of clinical nooks and crannies. Consider a doctor on his ward round, seeing patients. His junior doctor updates him on a particularly unwell patient with a serious infection, reeling off a string of blood test results. The doctor realises not only that the results remain outside the normal range, but also that they are worse than the day before. This deduction is a basic mathematical operation.

The doctor decides to switch the patient's antibiotic from an oral tablet to an intravenous infusion, knowing that this infusion is more likely to treat the infection. The antibiotic is potentially toxic in excess. The doctor double-checks the dose in his formulary and sees that the dose should be based on the patient's weight. The doctor looks up the patient's weight on his weight chart, calculates the required dose, and prescribes it for him.

This example is maths at work, saving lives.

The quantitative reasoning subtest is designed to assess how you solve numerical problems, some of which aren't dissimilar to those that we encounter in everyday clinical practice.

In this chapter, we show you everything you need to know to score highly in the UKCAT quantitative reasoning subtest. We include an explanation of the types of questions found in the quantitative reasoning subtest, some useful test strategies, and plenty of practice questions with answers and fully worked-through explanations.

Finding Out the Format of the Quantitative Reasoning Subtest

The UKCAT quantitative reasoning subtest typically consists of nine numerical presentations. After each presentation come four questions based on the content within the presentation, giving a total of 36 questions. The exact number of presentations and questions for each presentation can vary slightly, but the total number of questions is fixed at 36. You have 23 minutes to complete the subtest.

In the subtest, data is presented in the form of tables, charts and graphs. You have to be able to rapidly identify relevant information from the presentation, and then manipulate that information appropriately to answer the question.

The testers are looking for basic mathematical capabilities. They want to see that you can:

- ✔ Perform simple mathematical operations
- ✔ Understand proportions, percentages and ratios
- ✔ Apply different kinds of average
- ✔ Work comfortably with fractions and decimals
- ✔ Convert from one measurement system to another
- ✔ Solve basic equations

The UKCAT quantitative reasoning subtest focuses on using numbers to solve problems rather than on raw numerical facility. The subtest is checking that you can determine what numbers can reveal (and hide!), not whether you can number-crunch like a computer.

Most people find that, compared with the other sections of UKCAT, the quantitative reasoning subtest is intellectually simpler yet harder to complete within the time limit. Although the subtest is less conceptually difficult, try to remain focused throughout the subtest and don't let yourself make silly mathematical errors.

Since its most recent overhaul, the UKCAT prohibits the use of handheld calculators. The software used to administer the test includes an on-screen calculator with basic functionality. You can access this calculator with the click of an icon and let it run in the background as you move from one question to another. Many people find on-screen calculators harder to use than their more familiar handheld devices. To improve your familiarity with the on-screen calculator, try practising with the calculator program on most Windows PCs, and then do the practice tests on the UKCAT website to familiarise yourself with the real thing.

Preparing for Success in the Quantitative Reasoning Subtest

To do well in the quantitative reasoning subtest, you need to be familiar with some basic mathematical operations, which you may already be familiar with from GCSE-level mathematics:

- ✓ Addition, subtraction, multiplication and division
- ✓ Percentages, ratios and fractions
- ✓ Speed, distance and time calculations
- ✓ Working with money
- ✓ Areas and volumes
- ✓ Graphs and charts

If you feel you are rusty working with these simple operations, first have a look through your GCSE maths books again. Then get yourself up to speed by doing a lot of practice UKCAT questions.

Working Well on Test Day

Test day can be unnerving, making it easy to lose concentration and then panic. Add in the time pressure, and you may throw away scoring opportunities.

To help keep yourself focused, reduce your error rate and reduce your chances of spending too long on one question in the quantitative reasoning subtest, try to follow the tips below:

- ✓ **Try not to be intimidated by presentations on topics you know nothing about.** Remember that the testers are looking to see how well you can manipulate numerical information, not whether you're familiar with the topic of the presentation.

✔ **Practise using the on-screen calculator before test day.** Also, beware of typos when you use the on-screen calculator. On the day itself, try to leave yourself time to double-check the more complicated calculations.

✔ **Don't overcomplicate the questions.** The questions require the use of fairly basic mathematical operations. If you have to draw on advanced mathematics in your attempts to solve the problem, you're almost certainly overcomplicating things and heading down the wrong track.

✔ **If you're already comfortable working with maths, don't be overconfident in the subtest.** Read each question carefully and work steadily to avoid making careless errors. Vital information can easily be misinterpreted or missed entirely.

✔ **Don't relax too much.** Doing so leads to avoidable careless errors in a subtest that you can otherwise score highly on.

✔ **Don't spend too much time on a question you can't solve.** Move on to the next question and keep your cool.

The easiest way to understand these strategies is to practise questions, see how the answers are derived, and see how you can make mistakes if you lose concentration.

Practising Quantitative Reasoning

We suggest that you use this section to practise your quantitative reasoning skills. Concentrate on moving swiftly through the questions, avoiding careless and preventable errors. The content isn't mathematically challenging, provided you stay alert.

Don't be discouraged if you make a few mistakes. The whole point of this book is to prepare you for the actual test. Making a few mistakes now means you're less likely to make the same mistakes on test day.

Avoid rushing through this section. We include full sample tests for you to do under mock exam conditions in Part III. For now, concentrate on understanding the questions and answers and doing the best you can, even if you take a little more time than you have available in the real thing. Speed comes with practice and with increasing confidence.

EU Debt

The number of countries per group is shown in the figure.

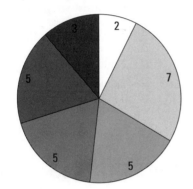

EU Countries Debt Burdens, expressed as a percentage of GDP and grouped by ranges

- □ >100%
- ▨ 80%-100%
- ▧ 60%-80%
- ▦ 40%-60%
- ▩ 20%-40%
- ■ <20%

1. To the nearest whole number, what percentage of countries have a debt greater than 100% of GDP?

A. 7%

B. 19%

C. 26%

D. 33%

E. 93%

2. What is the ratio of the number of countries with a debt burden greater than 80% of GDP to the rest of the countries?

A. 2:25

B. 1:2

C. 1:3

D. 8:27

E. 1:9

3. The countries with debts between 80% and 100% of GDP pass aggressive austerity budgets and as a result, three of them reduce their debts to between 60% and 80% of GDP. Assuming that all the other countries in the EU remain the same, what is the new ratio of countries with a debt burden greater than 80% of GDP to the rest of the countries?

A. 2:25
B. 5:22
C. 1:3
D. 6:21
E. 4:23

4. The EU countries in this survey account for a total of 500 million people. If the two countries with debts in excess of 100% of GDP account for 16% of that population, how many people live in each of the other countries, assuming that they're evenly distributed across the rest of the EU? Round your answer to the nearest whole million.

A. 6 million
B. 8 million
C. 17 million
D. 22 million
E. 40 million

Mental Health Act Assessments

The table shows the distribution of Mental Health Act assessments in 2010

Distribution of Mental Health Act Assessments in 2010	
Month	**Assessments**
January	132
February	85
March	88
April	101
May	95
June	110
July	123
August	117
September	78
October	92
November	167
December	286

5. How many assessments took place in the first three months of the year?

A. 132

B. 217

C. 305

D. 318

E. 406

6. By the end of which month had 50% of the assessments taken place?

A. May

B. June

C. July

D. August

E. September

7. What percentage of assessments, to the nearest whole number, took place in the last three months of the year?

A. 13%

B. 21%

C. 25%

D. 31%

E. 37%

8. The monitoring exercise was repeated a year later. The numbers of assessments had changed as follows: May (+15), June (−6), July (+7), August (−11). What's the new ratio of assessments in May and June to those in July and August, based on the revised totals?

A. 1:1

B. 113:129

C. 41:48

D. 107:118

E. 52:65

Medal-winning Performances

Mike, a football fan, decides to stratify the countries in the table immediately below into a league table of performance, shown in the second table.

2008 Olympic Gold Medals per Million Population					
Belarus	0.41	Slovenia	0.50	Spain	0.12
Jamaica	2.16	Great Britain	0.31	Italy	0.14
Portugal	0.09	Bahrain	1.41	Latvia	0.44
India	<0.01	Netherlands	0.42	Russia	0.16
Australia	0.69	Denmark	0.37	New Zealand	0.73
United States	0.12	Mongolia	0.68	Japan	0.07
Georgia	0.65	France	0.11	Norway	0.65

Country League Table

League	Number of Countries
Premiership (>1 gold per million)	2
Championship (0.7–0.99 gold per million)	1
League One (0.5–0.69 gold per million)	4
League Two (0.25–0.49 gold per million)	5
Conference (<0.25 gold per million)	8

9. What's wrong with Mike's table?

A. One too many in the Premiership

B. One too few in League One

C. One too few in League Two

D. One too many in the Conference

E. One too few in the Premiership

10. Great Britain has a population of 61.3 million. New Zealand has a population of 4.15 million. How many more gold medals did Great Britain win than New Zealand? Round your answer to the nearest whole medal.

A. 1

B. 2

C. 16

D. 25

E. 43

11. Mike is asked to calculate the modal average number of gold medals per million of the population. Which of the following should he do?

A. Find the gold-medal-per-million figure that occurs most frequently.

B. Add up all the gold-medal-per-million figures and divide by 21.

C. Add up all the gold-medal-per-million figures and divide by 2.

D. Rearrange the numbers into numerical order and find the tenth number.

E. Rearrange the numbers into numerical order, find the 10th and 11th numbers, add them up and divide by 2.

12. How many more gold medals would Great Britain have to win to achieve Championship status? (You may continue to assume that Great Britain has a population of 61.3 million.)

A. 12

B. 24

C. 31

D. 43

E. 61

Assessing UKCAT Scores

UKCAT Scores of Medical School Applicants

2,250	2,650	3,200 ·	2,900 ·	1,900
2,300	2,750 ·	2,400	3,050 ·	2,400
3,050 ·	2,150	2,800 ·	3,100 ·	2,900 ·
2,550	2,700	2,450	2,600	3,300 ·

13. Any applicant scoring 2,750 or greater is shortlisted for an interview. What percentage of applicants aren't called for an interview?

A. 35%

B. 40%

C. 45%

D. 55%

E. 60%

14. Based solely on the numbers in the table, what are any given applicant's odds of getting an interview? Round your answer to two decimal places.

A. 0.67

B. 0.82

C. 1.22

D. 1.5

E. 0.43

15. What proportion of applicants, expressed as a fraction, are interviewed if the cut-off score is 3,000?

A. $\frac{1}{5}$

B. $\frac{1}{4}$

C. $\frac{3}{10}$

D. $\frac{1}{20}$

E. $\frac{3}{4}$

16. What's the average UKCAT score of the interviewed candidates in the scenario outlined in question 15?

A. 3,140

B. 3,160

C. 3,180

D. 3,200

E. 3,240

Light Speed

Items 17–20 relate to faster-than-light (FTL) space travel.

Distance in space is measured in light years (lt-yr). One lt-yr is the distance covered by an object travelling at c, the speed of light, in 1 year. FTL speeds are measured by Warp factor. Warp factor is expressed as a multiple of c. Thus, Warp1 = c, Warp2 = $2c$, Warp3 = $3c$, Warp4 = $4c$ and so on. You may assume that 1 year = 365 days.

17. A spaceship leaves Earth in order to travel to the Alpha Centauri star system, 4.25 lt-yr away. Assuming travel at Warp5, how many days does it take to arrive at Alpha Centauri? Please express your answer in Earth days, and you may ignore any potential relativistic effects of FTL travel.

    A. 292.00
    B. 306.60
    C. 310.25
    D. 328.50
    E. 332.15

18. The spaceship's Warp drive requires frequent repairs. On the spaceship's journey to Alpha Centauri, it first breaks down after travelling 180 days at Warp6, and then again after 50 days at Warp4, before completing the rest of the journey at Warp7. How long did the last leg of the journey take, rounding your answer to the nearest whole day?

    A. 18
    B. 22
    C. 25
    D. 33
    E. 39

19. The spaceship runs on dilithium crystals and it takes 3 dilithium crystals to travel a light year. The spaceship is on a journey from Earth to a distant star system. The spaceship is currently 30% of the way from Earth to that distant system, and it has 21 further light years to travel before it reaches it. Before starting any journey, the ship's engineer always orders 10% extra dilithium crystals than the minimum needed for the trip. Assuming it is intended that the spaceship will return to Earth, how many crystals did the engineer order?

    A. 42
    B. 90
    C. 99
    D. 180
    E. 198

20. A wormhole is discovered between Earth and Alpha Centauri, which shortens the overall distance that needs to be travelled by a total 2 lt-yr. Travel through the wormhole is instantaneous. If a spaceship travels the 0.5 lt-yr to the wormhole at Warp2, and then travels at Warp5 from the wormhole to Alpha Centauri, how long is the total journey using the wormhole, expressed in days?

    A. 200.75
    B. 219.00
    C. 280.25
    D. 310.25
    E. 365.00

Governing Ruritania

The bars in the figure represent, in order, the votes for the Monarchist Party, the Rupertist Party, the Maubanite Party and other parties in the Ruritanian General Election, over five elections.

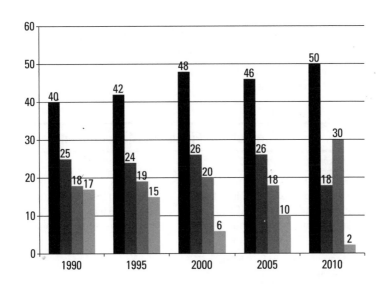

21. In 2005, what is the ratio of Rupertist votes to votes for all other parties?

A. 1:5

B. 1:4

C. 13:50

D. 13:37

E. 37:13

22. Which of the following statements is supported by the information in the chart?

A. The percentage of Rupertist votes is increasing over time.

B. The percentage of Maubanite votes is increasing over time.

C. The percentage vote for the Rupertists in 2005 is similar to that for the Maubanites in 1995.

D. The percentage of Monarchist votes has been increasing at the expense of Maubanites' votes.

E. The percentage of Monarchist votes has been increasing at the expense of Rupertists' and others' votes.

23. In 2010, 6.32 million people voted Monarchist. How many people voted Rupertist?

A. 9.50 million

B. 6.32 million

C. 3.60 million

D. 2.72 million

E. 2.28 million

24. What is the percentage range for all parties/groupings across the five elections?

A. 6%

B. 10%

C. 28%

D. 48%

E. 50%

Managing the Money Managers

The following tables show the charges levied by two different money management companies.

Wormtongue Financial Management

Portfolio set-up charge: £500			
Annual management fee (deducted on the anniversary date of portfolio creation)	Portfolio value of less than £50,000 on anniversary date	Portfolio value between £50,000 and £249,999 on anniversary date	Portfolio value greater than £250,000 on anniversary date
Percentage of portfolio value	0.5%	0.3%	0.1%

Thumbscrews Asset Management

Item	*Cost*
Portfolio set-up charge	Free
Annual management fee (deducted on the anniversary date of portfolio creation)	0.2% of portfolio value
Exit charge on money withdrawn from portfolio up to and including the first annual anniversary of set-up	0.08% of value of money withdrawn
Exit charge on money withdrawn from portfolio after first year	0.03% of value of money withdrawn

The questions in this section require some complicated calculations, although the mathematical operations involved are straightforward. The questions demonstrate how murky information can be when you want to compare tariffs between different providers. Similar kinds of calculation are required in real life when comparing mobile phone bills, mortgage providers and energy companies.

25. Josefin is looking for a wealth manager. She has narrowed her options down to these two firms. She has a lump sum of £200,000 to invest immediately and also plans to invest an extra £50,000 annually on the anniversary date of the portfolio's creation, for a further two years; that is, she will make two further payments into the portfolio.

These extra anniversary payments into the portfolio aren't included in the portfolio total when calculating fees owing on that same anniversary date, but do count towards future year totals.

Assuming that Josefin sticks to this schedule, how much will it cost her in overall fees and charges if she employs the services of Wormtongue Financial Management over her planned investment period (not including any fees that the portfolio attracts after the date of the final payment into the portfolio)?

You may assume that whatever funds are invested in the portfolio grow at 10% per year, and the annual management fees are deducted from Josefin's portfolio balance. Round your answer to the nearest penny.

A. £956.27

B. £1,456.27

C. £1,457.00

D. £1,700.00

E. £1,968.02

26. How much would Josefin's portfolio be worth if she invests the same amounts over the same timeframe as in question 25, but uses Thumbscrews Asset Management instead? Thumbscrews, like Wormtongue, generates a 10% annual growth rate.

A. £241,516.00

B. £295,922.97

C. £296,516.00

D. £345,922.97

E. £380,515.27

27. Josefin chooses to use Thumbscrews, and follows her investment plan as already outlined. However, she decides to withdraw the entire amount of her portfolio on the third anniversary of its set-up, in order to buy a house. How much does she pay Thumbscrews in exit charges?

A. £303.01

B. £284.56

C. £231.27

D. £143.63

E. £113.63

28. Which of the following statements is false?

A. If Josefin had less than £50,000 to invest overall, she would be best off using Thumbscrews.

B. If Josefin had £1,000,000 to invest for one year, she would be best off using Thumbscrews.

C. If Josefin had £1,000,000 to invest for one year, she would be best off using Wormtongue.

D. If Josefin wants to minimise her upfront costs, regardless of later charges, she is best off using Thumbscrews.

E. Thumbscrews penalise early withdrawals.

Death and Taxes

Numbers of Deaths in 2009 (in Thousands) from Different Causes

Cause of Death	Men	Women
Circulatory disease	78	82
Cancer	74	66
Respiratory disease	32	36
Digestive disease	12	13
Neurological disease	8	9
Mental disorder	6	12
Genitourinary disease	5	7
Endocrine disease	3	4
Infectious disease	2	3

29. What is the average number of deaths, in thousands and to the nearest thousand, across all the causes of death in men?

    A. 78
    B. 32
    C. 44
    D. 24
    E. 22

30. Find the difference between men's and women's deaths due to digestive disease or mental disorder and express this difference as a percentage of men's deaths from those conditions.

    A. 8.3%
    B. 28%
    C. 33.3%
    D. 38.9%
    E. 50.0%

31. What is the difference, in thousands of deaths, between the fifth most common cause of death for men and the fifth most common cause of death for women?

    A. 0
    B. 1
    C. 4
    D. 8
    E. 10

32. Which of the following statements is true?

    A. Men more commonly die of mental disorder than women do.
    B. More women than men die of circulatory disease.
    C. More women than men die of cancer.
    D. Infectious disease is the least common cause of death in men, but only the second least common in women.
    E. The number of people who die of respiratory disease is greater than the number of women who die from circulatory disease.

Changing Rooms

Mr Wickes has decided to convert his master bathroom into a wet room. This decision means that the entire floor and walls have to be waterproofed and then tiled up to the ceiling, and a central drain has to be fitted to the floor.

For the purposes of this question, the bathroom can be considered to have a simple cuboidal structure, as pictured below.

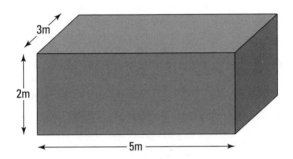

33. Waterproofing costs £8 per 0.75 square metres to be covered. Travertine tiles cost £70 per square metre. How much will it cost, in terms of materials, to waterproof and tile the new wet room, to the nearest hundred pounds?

A. £1,100
B. £2,600
C. £3,300
D. £3,800
E. £4,200

34. Waterproofing takes 10 minutes per square metre, and tiling takes 2 hours per square metre. How long will it take to complete the job, to the nearest hour?

A. 64 hours
B. 94 hours
C. 102 hours
D. 104 hours
E. 124 hours

35. Mr Wickes breaks the habit of a lifetime and decides not to do the job himself. Instead, he hires a professional tiler, who charges £12 an hour as well as charging Mr Wickes the full market rate for the materials required. Assuming the tiler can access the materials at a 20% trade discount, how much profit does he make from the job, to the nearest £100?

A. £1,200

B. £2,000

C. £3,600

D. £4,300

E. £5,000

36. Mr Wickes decides to buy a new shower system for his wet room. He goes for a thermostatic body jet shower mixer which costs £400. It pumps out approximately 12 litres of water per minute. Mr Wickes' water company charges £2 per cubic metre of water. Assuming he uses his new shower for 15 minutes per day, how much does the shower cost him annually, over a five-year period, if he evenly amortises the capital cost of the shower system over that time-frame? Do not consider any of the other wet-room costs. Assume that each year is 365 days long and that Mr Wickes never goes on holiday.

A. £131.40

B. £211.40

C. £631.40

D. £657.00

E. £1,057.00

Answers

1. A: 7%

   Two countries have a debt greater than 10% of GDP. The survey includes 27 countries. $(2/17) \times 100 = 7\%$ to the nearest whole number.

2. B: 1:2.

   Nine countries have a debt greater than 80%. The survey includes 27 countries; therefore, 18 other countries are in the EU. The ratio is 9:18, which simplifies to 1:2.

3. D: 6:21

   Seven countries are in the range of 80–100%. If three of these countries succeed in moving into the range of 60–80% as a result of their austerity measures, four countries remain in the range of 60–80%. Including the two countries with debts above 100%, a total of six countries now have debts greater than 80%. As the total number of countries is 27, the ratio of countries with debts above 80% to those below is 6:21.

4. C: 17 million

   The total population is 500 million. The two countries with debts above 100% of GDP account for 16% of the population, which in terms of millions of people is 500 million $\times$ (16 $\div$ 100) = 80 million. Therefore, the remaining 25 countries account for (500 – 80) = 420 million people.

   You're told that the remaining population is distributed evenly across those 25 countries, so the number of people in each country is 420 $\div$ 25 million = 17 million, to the nearest whole number.

5. C: 305

   This test is a straightforward check of your ability to extract the relevant data from the table and then add the numbers together to find the total. The relevant data for the answer is included in this table.

Assessments in the First Three Months	
Month	*Assessments*
January	132
February	85
March	88

   132 + 85 + 88 = 305.

6. D: August.

   Solving this problem is a two-step operation. First you need to find 50% of the total number of assessments. The total is 1,474 (calculated by adding up each of the individual data points). The 50% mark is therefore 737 assessments.

   Then work your way down the table, adding up the assessments as you go, until you go past 737. This point occurs after you pass August, so the answer is D.

7. E: 37%

   First you need to find the total number of assessments that took place in the last three months of the year. Take a look at the relevant information in this table.

Assessments in the Last Three Months

Month	Assessments
October	92
November	167
December	286

   92 + 167 + 286 = 545.

   As the total number of assessments is 1,474 (which you calculated for Item 6), the percentage is $545 \div 1{,}474 \times 100 = 37\%$ to the nearest whole number.

8. D: 107:118

   You've been given the change in data compared with the earlier year. You can quickly determine the new totals, outlined in this table.

New Distribution of Assessments in 2011

Month	Assessments
May	95 + 15 = 110
June	110 − 6 = 104
July	123 + 7 = 130
August	117 − 11 = 106

To work out the ratio between the months of May and June and July and August, you need to add up the relevant data points:

May + June = 110 + 104 = 214

July + August = 130 + 106 = 236

The ratio 214:236 simplifies to 107:118.

9. B: One too few in League One.

The relevant League One countries are highlighted in bold in the following table. Five countries are highlighted, but only four countries are counted in the Country League table. Answering this question requires that you do the same task Mike attempted and check your totals against his as you go.

League One Countries					
Belarus	0.41	**Slovenia**	**0.50**	Spain	0.12
Jamaica	2.16	Great Britain	0.31	Italy	0.14
Portugal	0.09	Bahrain	1.41	Latvia	0.44
India	<0.01	Netherlands	0.42	Russia	0.16
Australia	**0.69**	Denmark	0.37	New Zealand	0.73
United States	0.12	**Mongolia**	**0.68**	Japan	0.07
Georgia	**0.65**	France	0.11	**Norway**	**0.65**

10. C: 16.

This question involves a multi-stage calculation. The data in Table 5-2 shows gold medals per country per million population. Before calculating the difference, you have to convert these standardised figures back into absolute numbers of gold medals won by Great Britain and New Zealand by multiplying each figure by its population:

Number of gold medals won by Great Britain = 0.31 × 61.3 = 19 medals, to the nearest whole number.

Number of gold medals won by New Zealand = 0.73 × 4.15 = 3 medals, again to the nearest whole number.

Then you subtract the British total from the New Zealand total = 19 – 3 = 16.

11. A: Find the gold-medal-per million figure that occurs most frequently.

    This question checks that you understand the term 'modal average'.

12. B: 24

    To be in the Championship, Great Britain needs a minimum gold medal per million of 0.7. As its population size is 61.3, Great Britain needs to win 61.3 × 0.7 = 43 medals (rounding up to the nearest whole gold medal). You've already calculated that Great Britain has won 19 medals, so it needs to win 43 – 19 = 24 more gold medals.

13. D: 55%

    Nine applicants have a score of 2,750 or greater. As Table 5-4 shows scores for a total of 20 candidates, 20 – 9 = 11 candidates were not selected for interview. Expressed as a percentage, this calculation is (11 ÷ 20) × 100 = 55%.

14. B: 0.82

    Odds are expressed as the number of chances of an event happening compared with the number of chances of the same event not happening. The question lists 9 interviewed candidates and 11 non-interviewed candidates, so the odds of being interviewed are 9:11, or 9/11, or in decimal form 0.82.

15. B: ¼

    Only 5 applicants out of a total of 20 have scores of 3,000 or above. Expressed as a fraction, this calculation is 5 ÷ 20 = ¼.

16. A: 3,140

    This question is a straightforward test of your ability to calculate an arithmetic mean, in this case of the five candidates with scores of 3,000 or above: (3,200 + 3,050 + 3,050 + 3,100 + 3,300) ÷ 5 = 3,140.

17. C: 310.25

    Questions 17–20 involve topics that are partly the realm of science fiction and partly the realm of quantum physics. The mathematics you're required to do in order to answer the questions, however, is straightforward. Don't be fazed by unusual topics – just focus on the maths!

    The key thing to realise for this set of questions is that if distance is expressed in light years (with 1 lt-yr being the distance covered by light in a year) and Warp speeds are multiples of the speed of light, then dividing any distance in light years by a Warp speed gives you an answer in years. So, the time for any journey (in years) can be found by dividing light years by Warp factor. All the information required to work this out is within the question, with no mathematics more complicated than GCSE-level knowledge and no knowledge of physics required.

The distance to Alpha Centauri is 4.25 lt-yr. The spaceship is travelling at Warp5, which is $5c$. In 1 year, the spaceship will cover 5 lt-yr (because c is the speed of light).

Time = distance ÷ speed = 4.25 ÷ 5 = 0.85 years

As a year has 365 days, the spaceship takes 0.85 × 365 = 310.25 days to reach Alpha Centauri.

18. E: 39

This question involves a fairly complicated multi-stage calculation. You know that the total distance to be travelled is 4.25 lt-yr. To calculate how long the last leg took, you need to calculate the distance left to travel during that leg. You know the speed the spaceship travelled at, so you can work out how long the final leg took.

To calculate the distance of the final leg, you work out the distances of the first two legs, add them together, and then subtract them from the total journey distance. You already know the speed of the first two legs and the time in days (which you can easily convert to time in years). You need to use the equation distance = speed × time:

First leg: $6c$ × (180 ÷ 365) = 2.96 lt-yr

Second leg: $4c$ × (50 ÷ 365) = 0.55 lt-yr

Distance of third leg = 4.25 − 2.96 − 0.55 = 0.74 lt-yr

The time in days to cover the third leg = distance ÷ speed = (0.74 ÷ $7c$) × 365 = 39 days (multiplying by 365 to convert from years into days, and then rounding to the nearest whole day).

19. E: 198

The spaceship has 21 lt-yr left to travel to its destination, and has already travelled 30% of the trip to the star system. This means that 21 lt-yr represents 70% of the total distance between Earth and the destination. The total distance is (100 ÷ 70) × 21 = 30 lt-yr.

Because the spaceship will make a return journey, the total distance is 30 × 2 = 60 lt-yr.

At a consumption rate of 3 crystals per lt-yr, the minimum number of crystals required is 60 × 3 = 180 crystals. Adding in the engineer's 10% safety buffer gives: (110 ÷ 100) × 180 = 198 crystals.

20. B: 219

The original distance from Earth to Alpha Centauri is 4.25 lt-yr. The wormhole shortens travel by 2 lt-yr, so the new total distance is 2.25 lt-yr.

The journey to the wormhole is 0.5 lt-yr, so the journey from the wormhole is 2.25 − 0.5 = 1.75 lt-yr.

Time to reach the wormhole = distance ÷ speed = 0.5 ÷ 2 = 0.25 years

Time from the wormhole to Alpha Centauri = distance ÷ speed = 1.75 ÷ 5 = 0.35 years

The total journey time is 0.25 + 0.35 = 0.6 years. Converting into days, this calculation is 0.6 × 365 = 219 days.

21. D: 13:37

In all, 26% voted Rupertist and 74% voted for other parties. The ratio is 26:74, which simplifies to 13:37.

22. B: The percentage of Maubanite votes is increasing over time.

You can see this information relatively easily in the chart. The other options are contrary to the information provided or incomplete assumptions.

23. E: 2.28m

A total of 6.32 million people account for 50% of votes cast. Therefore, the total number of votes cast is 6.32 × (100/50) = 12.64 million.

18% of votes cast were Rupertist votes. Therefore, the number of Rupertist votes is 12.64 million × 0.18 = 2.28 million.

If you're comfortable with maths, a quicker method is to calculate 18 ÷ 50 × 6.32, making use of the relative proportions of the Monarchist and Rupertist parties.

24. D: 48%

The range is the highest reading across the period minus the lowest reading across the period = 50% − 2% = 48%.

25. B: £1,456.27

Wormtongue charges a portfolio set-up fee of £500, which must be added to any other charges. The company also charges an annual management fee, which is based on a percentage of the total funds being managed, with a discounted rate for larger portfolios. Remember also that Josefin's fund grows in size by 10% every year because of the investments that Wormtongue makes with her money.

The fees for Josefin are shown in bold in the calculations below:

Portfolio creation: **£500** set-up fee

Year-one anniversary portfolio value: £200,000 × 110 ÷ 100 = £220,000

Year-one fee: £220,000 × 0.3% = **£660**

Year-one balance: £220,000 − £660 = £219,340

Add Josefin's new £50,000 investment: £219,340 + £50,000 = £269,340

Year-two anniversary portfolio balance: £269,340 × 110 ÷ 100 = £296,274

Year-two fee: £296,274 × 0.1% = **£296.27**

Year-two balance: £296,274 − £296.74 = £295,977.73

Add Josefin's new £50,000 investment = £295,977.73 + £50,000 = £345,977.73

The total fees are therefore £500 + £660 + £296.27 = **£1,456.27**

26. D: £345,922.97

   The calculation can be broken down as follows:

   Portfolio creation: free

   Year-one anniversary portfolio value: £200,000 × 110 ÷ 100 = £220,000

   Year-one fee: £220,000 × 0.2% = £440

   Year-one balance: £220,000 − £440 = £219,560

   Add Josefin's new £50,000 investment: £219,560 + £50,000 = £269,560

   Year-two anniversary portfolio value = £269,560 × 110 ÷ 100 = £296,516

   Year-two fee: £296,516 × 0.2% = £593.03

   Year-two balance: £296,516 − £593.03 = £295,922.97

   Add Josefin's new £50,000 investment: £295,922.97 + £50,000 = £345,922.97

Despite the different fee structures between the two companies, the fund grows to pretty much the same size with both firms. This kind of thing often happens in real life too.

27. E – £113.63

    Extending the calculation from Answer 26:

    Year-three anniversary portfolio value = £345,022.97 × 110 – 100 = £379,525.27

    Year-three fee: £379,525.27 × 0.2% = £759.05

    Year-three balance: £379,525.27 – £759.05 = £378,766.22

    Exit charge = £378,766.22 × 0.03% = £113.63

28. B: If Josefin had £1,000,000 to invest for one year, she would be best off using Thumbscrews.

    You can solve this question by working through all the options. Answer B is clearly false, because Wormtongue charge 0.1% per annum for large portfolios, compared with Thumbscrews' 0.2% flat rate. Even the £500 set-up fee that Wormtongue charges cannot possibly outweigh the percentage difference for such a large balance, even without considering the percentage-based exit charge that Thumbscrews adds too.

29. D: 24

    This question is a straightforward test of your ability to work out the arithmetic mean of all the data points in the 'Men' column. The sum is 78 + 74 + 32 + 12 + 8 + 6 + 5 + 3 + 2 = 220. The mean is 220 ÷ 9 = 24.4 to one decimal place, or 24 to the nearest thousand.

30. D: 38.9%

    A total of 12 + 6 = 18 thousand men died from digestive and mental disorders combined. A total of 13 + 12 = 25 thousand women died from the two causes combined. So 25 – 18 = 7 thousand more women died than men.

    Expressed as a percentage compared with the number of men that died, the answer is (7 ÷ 18) × 100 = 38.9%.

31. C: 4

    The fifth most common cause of death in men is neurological disease, with 8,000 deaths. The fifth most common cause of death in women is mental disorder, with 12,000. The difference is 4,000 deaths, or 4 if expressed in thousands.

    This question tests your ability to note that although Table 5-7 is sorted by frequency of death in men, women's causes of death don't share the same order, so the fifth most common cause of death in men is different from that in women.

32. B: More women than men die of circulatory disease.

This question is relatively straightforward. You can find the answer simply by testing each statement's truth against the data in Table 5-7.

33. D: £3,800

First you need to calculate the area to be waterproofed and tiled. This area consists of the four walls and the floor:

Wall area = [2 × (2 × 5)] + [2 × (2 × 3)] = 20 + 12 = 32 square metres

Floor area = 3 × 5 = 15 square metres

Total area = 32 + 15 = 47 square metres to be waterproofed and tiled

Waterproofing costs = (47 ÷ 0.75) × 8 = £501.33

Tiling costs = 47 × 70 = £3,290

The total cost is £501.33 + £3,290 = £3,791.33, or £3,800 to the nearest hundred pounds.

Mr Wickes needs to tile the floor but not the ceiling. Also, don't forget to include the waterproofing costs in your answer.

34. C: 102 hours

From Answer 33 you already know the area to be worked on: 47 square metres. If waterproofing takes 10 minutes per square metre, waterproofing takes (47 × 10) ÷ 60 = 7.83 hours to two decimal places. Tiling takes 2 hours per square metre, for a total of 47 × 2 = 94 hours.

The total time is approximately (because the above answer is inexact) 7.83 + 94 = 101.83, or 102 hours to the nearest hour.

35. B: £2,000

From Answer 34 you already know that the job takes 102 hours, which at £12 per hour comes to a labour charge of £1,224. You already know that the materials cost £3,800, but the tiler buys them at a 20% discount, so he makes a further profit of £3,800 × 0.2 = £760 on materials.

The tiler therefore makes a total profit of £1,224 + £760 = £1,984, or £2,000 to the nearest hundred.

Incidentally, the figures in this question aren't entirely unrealistic, which means that if the tiler has enough work to keep him busy full-time, he can earn well north of £40,000 a year, and possibly significantly more in better economic times, when he can charge somewhere in the region of £20 per hour. Of course, he still has to cover any other business expenses and pay his taxes after this!

36. B: £211.40

The shower uses 12 litres per minute and runs for 15 minutes per day, 365 days per year. The total annual water usage is therefore $12 \times 15 \times 365 = 65{,}700$ litres, or 65.7 cubic metres. At a cost of £2 per cubic metre, the annual cost of water is $65.7 \times £2 = £131.4$.

The shower itself costs £400, which you have to amortise over a 5-year period. Each year, therefore, the shower costs the equivalent of $£400 \div 5 = £80$. Adding this amount to the water costs, $£131.4 + £80 = £211.40$.

Chapter 6

Looking at Pretty Patterns: The Abstract Reasoning Subtest

*T*he abstract reasoning subtest is odd. We can think of no other way to describe this subtest.

In the test, you look at groups of strange pictures and identify how the pictures are related to each other. You then either work out which group the next item in the list belongs to, or what item comes next in the series.

The abstract reasoning subtest assesses how you infer relationships from the patterns of abstract shapes. The patterns may include irrelevant and distracting material, which the examiners include as a *red herring,* sometimes leading you to give the wrong answer.

Many students find this section of the UKCAT the most intimidating. Whereas the verbal and quantitative reasoning subtests deal with familiar concepts, the abstract reasoning subtest is . . . well . . . abstract.

To understand why a test for prospective doctors and dentists includes something so abstract, consider a dentist about to see a patient in her clinic.

As the patient relates his medical history, the dentist part listens and part thinks. She looks ahead, formulating hypotheses as to what may be wrong with the patient and deciding what questions she needs to ask to prove or disprove her hypotheses. Working in this way keeps the consultation brief but productive, and lets the dentist concentrate on helping the patient understand what's going on rather than pestering him with endless questions.

The dentist's way of working feels instinctive to her, but it's actually the product of a lot of training, accumulation of knowledge, and ability to apply *pattern recognition* – that is, to identify thematic similarities between the patient in the chair and patients she's seen in the past. Those similarities help her form an idea of what the patient is suffering from, even before looking in his mouth. As the patient divulges more information, the dentist slots the data into her overall impression, narrowing down the options to obtain the correct diagnosis.

Training has helped the dentist in this task, but the job's much easier if she's naturally talented at this sort of thing. The UKCAT abstract reasoning subtest measures this natural ability.

To be successful in this subtest, you need to demonstrate a scientific approach to recognising patterns. You need to rapidly create hypotheses, test them against the available information, and use the results to generate answers.

In this chapter, we offer all you need to score highly in the UKCAT abstract reasoning subtest. We include an explanation of the types of question found in the subtest, some useful test strategies and plenty of practice questions, with answers and fully worked-through explanations.

Figuring Out the Format of the Abstract Reasoning Subtest

This subtest includes four different types of question:

- ✔ Type 1: You see two sets of shapes, labelled Set A and Set B. The shapes in Set A all have something in common about their patterns. Likewise, all the shapes in Set B have something in common about their patterns. The two sets of shapes aren't related to each other in any way. For each pair of sets, you then see five test shapes. Your task is to decide whether each test shape belongs to Set A, Set B or neither.

- ✔ Type 2: You see a series of shapes where each shape is related to the previous one in the series by a consistent rule. You work out the rule so you can select the next item in the series from a choice of potential answer shapes.

- ✔ Type 3: The test tells you that two shapes are related but does not explain how. It also shows you a third shape. You decide what shape, from a selection of possible answer shapes, relates to the third shape in the same way as the first two shapes are related.

- ✔ Type 4: You see two sets of shapes, labelled Set A and Set B. You then decide which of four answer shapes fits into a specified set.

The subtest contains 55 questions. You have just 14 minutes to complete the subtest.

To answer 55 questions in 14 minutes, you need to work very fast: at a rate of about 4 questions a minute.

Working Out Patterns in the Abstract Reasoning Subtest

The four types of question appear very different but test the same basic skill of spotting underlying patterns and relationships. Sometimes the similarity or progression rule is instantly obvious. Certain relationships and rules tend to appear frequently in this subtest, so familiarity and practice increase the chance of quickly being able to spot the pattern.

At other times, however, the relationship is harder to spot. This is especially true if it's a complex rule with more than one element. For example, if the similarities relate both to the number of sides of an object within a shape and to its colour, and you only spot one of the rules (say the one about colour), you'll still find it hard to answer the question.

To gain time and score highly, we suggest that you use a systematic common approach to identifying similarities within a set, or progression rules within a series. This approach should become second nature, and can be exercised on any question without an obvious solution.

With practice, you discover your own best approach to answering questions in the abstract reasoning subtest, but for now try working through the following list of ideas to focus quickly on the commonality within each set or the progression within a series:

- Shape of components
- Number of corners on each component
- Type of edges on each component
- Colour of each component
- Number of components
- Orientation of components
- Consistent (or consistently evolving) position of one component relative to the others
- Size of components

By applying this list of possible similarities to each set, you can quickly generate potential hypotheses about the set. You can then test each hypothesis in turn, accepting or discarding hypotheses as applicable.

The list above isn't exhaustive. Also, sometimes more than one rule applies, making the question more complicated. But our suggestions are a good starting point and may get you out of trouble if you're stuck on a question.

The more abstract reasoning questions you practise, the easier you'll find this subtest.

Coping With the Abstract Reasoning Subtest on Test Day

The abstract reasoning subtest is intimidating. Many candidates panic and give up too quickly, which is understandable because you need to answer four questions a minute to complete the subtest. Try using the tips below to help you keep your cool:

- **Don't be intimidated by a set or series you can't solve instantly.** Consider the list of basic commonalities and work your way through each possibility. If none of the possibilities fits the set of shapes, move on to the next question. You can always come back to a set later on. By keeping moving, you maximise your scoring opportunities.

- **Remember that you have more time than you think.** The time-consuming portion of the subtest is identifying the commonality in the first place – try to think in terms of time per set rather than time per question. After you spot the commonality in a set, seeing which set each test shape belongs to is usually quick and easy.

- **Accept that some sets are complex.** The sets towards the end of the subtest are particularly complicated, with multiple interacting features. Few candidates solve these questions, so don't be surprised if you can't.

- **Be wary of red herrings.** Look out for features that appear to present the solution but aren't quite correct. Check your answer. If your answer's correct, you'll find no exceptions to the commonality rule within a set and you'll see a consistent difference between the sets.

- **If you feel that you've done badly in the subtest, take a few deep breaths and try to mentally set the test aside.** The UKCAT tests a range of different aptitudes, and few people excel at all of them. Try to refocus on maximising your score on the next subtest.

The easiest way to understand how these strategies work in practice is to do some questions, see how the answers are derived, and see how easy the questions are when you spot the commonality quickly.

Practising Abstract Reasoning

In this section, we give you many questions to help you practise your abstract reasoning skills. We include 55 items in total, just like in the real UKCAT test. Concentrate on moving swiftly through the questions.

To which set, if either, does each of the test shapes (Q1 to Q5) belong?

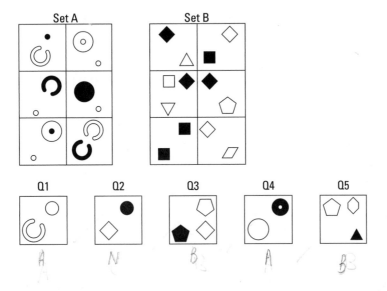

To which set, if either, does each of the test shapes (Q6 to Q10) belong?

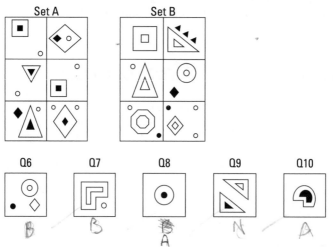

To which set, if either, does each of the test shapes (Q11 to Q15) belong?

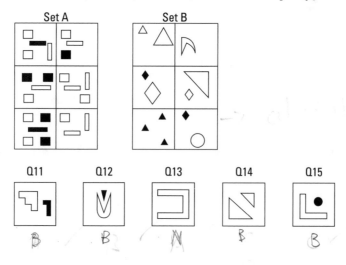

16. Which figure completes the series?

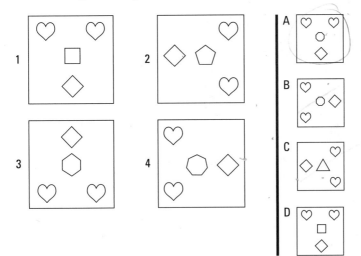

17. Which figure completes the series?

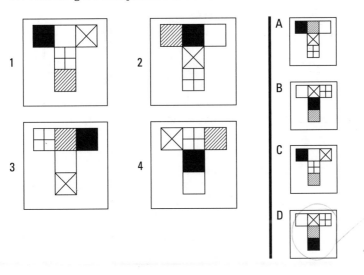

18. Which figure completes the statement?

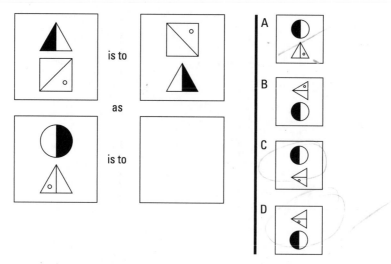

19. Which of the test shapes belongs to Set A?

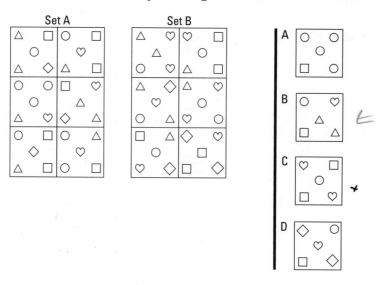

20. Which of the test shapes belongs to Set B?

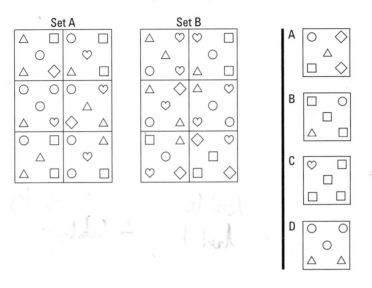

To which set, if either, does each of the test shapes (Q21 to Q25) belong?

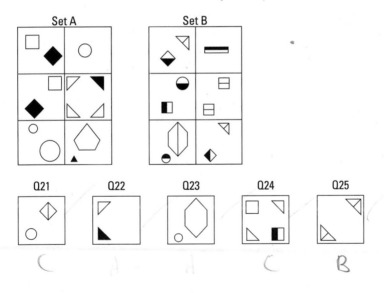

To which set, if either, does each of the test shapes (Q26 to Q30) belong?

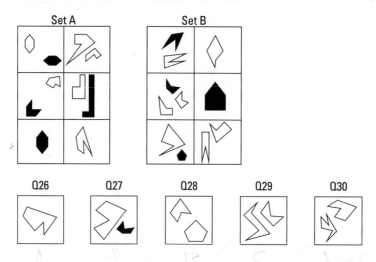

31. Which figure completes the statement?

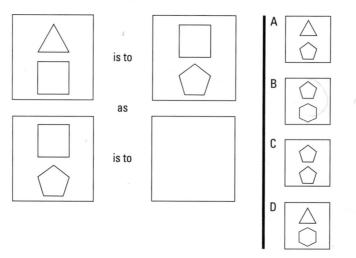

32. Which figure completes the statement?

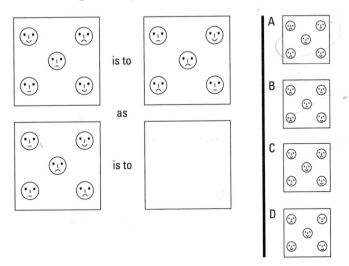

33. Which figure completes the series?

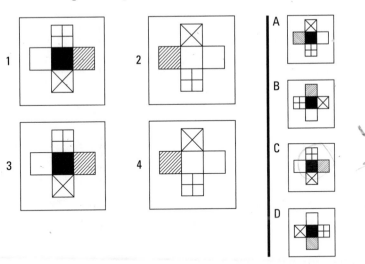

34. Which of the test shapes (A to D) belongs to Set A?

Set A 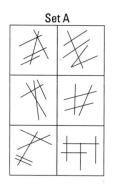 Set B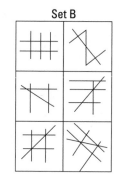

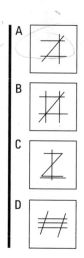

35. Which of the test shapes (A to D) belongs to Set B?

Set A 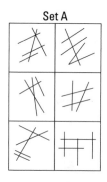 Set B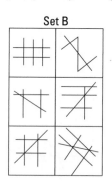

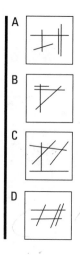

To which set, if either, does each of the test shapes (Q36 to Q40) belong?

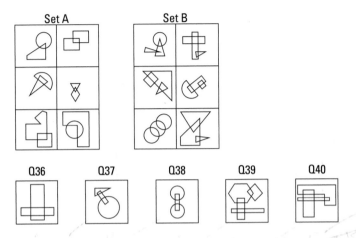

To which set, if either, does each of the test shapes (Q41 to Q45) belong?

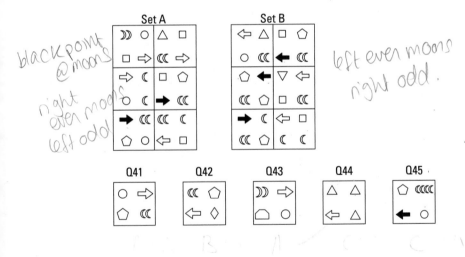

46. Which of the test shapes (A to D) belongs to Set A?

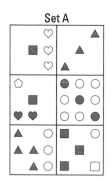

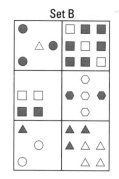

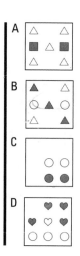

47. Which of the test shapes (A to D) belongs to Set B?

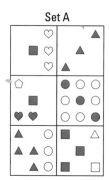

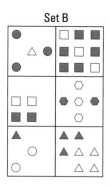

48. Which of the test shapes (A to D) completes the statement?

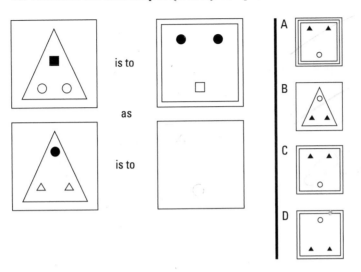

49. Which of the test shapes (A to D) completes the statement?

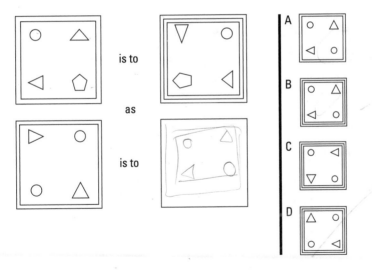

50. Which of the test shapes (A to D) completes the series?

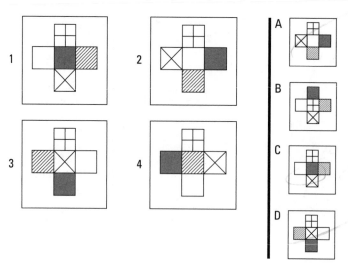

To which set, if either, does each of the test shapes (Q51 to Q55) belong?

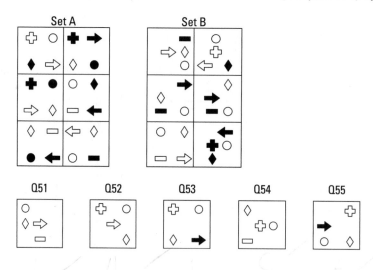

Answers

1, Set A; **2**, neither set; **3**, Set B; **4**, Set A; **5**, Set B

Explanation

All the shapes in Set A have curved edges. All the shapes in Set B have straight edges. The size, colour and orientation of the shapes demonstrate no commonality within the sets.

Test shapes 1 and 4 contain only shapes with curved edges and therefore fall into Set A. Test shapes 3 and 5 contain only shapes with straight edges and so fall into Set B. Test shape 2 contains shapes with both curved and straight edges and therefore doesn't go in either set.

6, Set B; **7**, Set B; **8**, Set A; **9**, neither set; **10**, Set A

Explanation

All the examples in Set A contain a shape that's internally replicated with a shape of the opposite colour. For instance, the top-left item contains a large white square with a smaller black inner square, while the top-right item contains a large white rhombus with a smaller black inner rhombus.

All the examples in Set B contain a shape that's internally replicated with a shape of the same colour. For instance, the top-left item contains a large square with a smaller white inner square, while the top-right item contains a large white right-angled triangle with a smaller white right-angled triangle within it.

Apart from this, the placement and orientation of the large object within the box are irrelevant, and any other shapes featured in each item show no consistent features of commonality.

Test shapes 6 and 7 contain a large object that is replicated internally by a smaller white item, and so both fall within Set B. Test shapes 8 and 10 contain a large object that is internally replicated with a smaller white object, and so both fit in Set A. Test shape 9 has both types of internal replication and so falls into neither set.

11, Set A; **12**, Set B; **13**, Set A; **14**, Set B; **15**, neither set

Explanation

All the examples in Set A contain items that have at least two right-angles each. All the examples in Set B contain items that have at most one right-angle each. The exact nature of the overall shape, the colour and the orientation show no consistent features of commonality.

Test shapes 11 and 13 have only objects with at least two right-angles and so fit in Set A. Test shapes 12 and 14 have only objects with at most one right-angle each and so fall within Set B. Test shape 15 has one object with four right-angles, but also a shape with no right-angles, therefore it can't be classified as Set A or Set B.

16, A

Explanation

The peripheral hearts and diamond rotate by 90 degrees clockwise each time. At the same time, the number of sides in the central figure increases by one.

17, D

Explanation

The lowest square moves up to the top left, displacing the top left square to the right. The top right square is in turn displaced further down.

18, D

Explanation

The top shape shifts to the bottom, and the white and black areas are reversed. The bottom shape shifts to the top and rotates by 90 degrees anticlockwise.

19, B; **20**, C

Explanation

All the boxes in Set A contain at least one equilateral triangle. All the boxes in Set B contain at least one heart.

21, neither set; **22**, Set A; **23**, Set A; **24**, neither set; **25**, Set B

Explanation

All the objects in Set A have no internal subdivisions. All the objects in Set B have internal subdivisions. The exact nature of the overall shape, the colour of the shapes and subdivisions, and the orientation show no consistent features of commonality.

Test shapes 22 and 23 have only objects without subdivisions and are therefore members of Set A. Test shape 25 contains only objects with subdivisions and is therefore a member of Set B. Test shapes 21 and 24 has a mix of objects with and without subdivisions, and so can't be classified into either set.

26, Set A; **27**, Set A; **28**, Set B; **29**, neither set; **30**, neither set

Explanation

All the objects in Set A are six sided. All the objects in Set B are five-sided. The colour of the shapes and their orientations show no consistent features of commonality.

Test shapes 26 and 27 contain only six-sided objects and so fall within Set A. Test shape 28 contains only five-sided objects and so is in Set B. Test shapes 29 and 30 contain objects with various numbers of sides and so don't fall within either set.

31, B

Explanation

Each shape gains one side.

32, A

Explanation

Happy faces become straight faces, sad faces become happy faces, and straight faces become sad faces.

33, C

Explanation

The middle square alternates from black to white. Peripherally, the right and left squares swap places, as do the top and bottom squares. There is no simple rotation.

34, A; **35**, D

Explanation

In Set A, the lines always create one enclosed space. In Set B, the lines always create two enclosed spaces.

36, Set A; **37**, Set B; **38**, Set B; **39**, neither set; **40**, neither set

Explanation

Set A contains objects that form only one overlapping area. Set B contains objects that form two areas of overlap.

Whenever you see objects that intersect with each other, consider whether the number of overlapping areas, or the colour or shape of the overlapping area, forms a set commonality. In this set, the number of overlaps is a commonality.

Test shape 36 has one area of overlap and so falls within Set A. Test shapes 37 and 38 both contain two areas of overlap and so are members of Set B. Test shapes 39 and 40 both contain three areas of overlap and so fall into neither set.

Don't be tempted to overcomplicate the solution – this subtest is confusing enough already! You may argue that the Set B commonality is 'at least two areas of overlap' rather than simply 'two areas of overlap'. You may also argue that it is the number of shapes rather than the number of areas of overlap that matters. In potentially ambiguous cases, you must apply Occam's razor. This is the logical principle that if more than one solution can apply, the simplest solution is usually the correct one. This is used often in medical and dental fields to narrow down a broad differential diagnosis, and is best summarised by the truism: 'Common things are common.' Health professionals who jump to an obscure and rare diagnosis when faced with common symptoms are sometimes whimsically referred to as 'hunting for zebras'. Horses are more common, at least in European and North American practice! No object in Set B contains more than two areas of overlap, so the most logical commonality is 'two areas of overlap' rather than 'at least two areas of overlap'. If the elements are depicted as overlapping, whereas in most other parts of the abstract reasoning subtest they are depicted discretely (alone), then it's wise to focus on the overlap rather than on anything else.

41, neither set; **42**, neither set; **43**, Set A; **44**, Set A; **45**, Set A

Explanation

This question takes the abstract reasoning subtest to the next level. Instead of examining individual objects, you have to consider the relationship of one object to other objects within the same shape.

A clue that you need to head down this complicated route is if you see objects that point in one direction and then change direction between shapes. Objects such as arrows and triangles are classic examples. Also look for objects that appear consistently between shapes but change colour from one shape to the next.

In Set A, if you see exactly two crescent moons, the arrow points right. With any other number of moons, the arrow points left. In addition, if you see a pentagon, the arrow is black.

In Set B, if you see exactly two crescent moons, the arrow points left. With any other number of moons, the arrow points right. In addition, if you see a pentagon, the arrow is black.

The pentagon-related colour change doesn't let you differentiate between the two sets, but you can use the colour change to determine whether shapes fit into either set at all. The orientation of the arrow in response to the number of crescent moons is diagnostic.

Test shape 41 has two crescent moons and a right-pointing arrow; however, the shape has a pentagon but the arrow is white instead of black, and so it doesn't fit in either set. Test shape 42 has a similar issue, forcing it out of both sets.

Test shape 43 has two crescent moons and a right-pointing arrow. No pentagon means that the shape is correctly coloured white, so the shape falls into Set A. Test shapes 44 and 45 don't have two moons and have left-pointing arrows, fitting with Set A; you can confirm this by noticing the correct colour for their respective pentagon status.

46, B; **47**, C

Explanation

In Set A, the central shape is always black; in Set B it is always white.

48, C

Explanation

The large triangle changes to a square (with a single border). The small shapes within the triangle rotate by 180 degrees, and those that were white become black and vice versa.

49, B

Explanation

The large square gains another border. Meanwhile, the smaller figures within the large square rotate by 90 degrees clockwise for position, and 90 degrees anticlockwise in orientation.

50, C

Explanation

The cross in the top square is stationary. Meanwhile, the four other squares keep on moving one across, with the right-most square falling to the bottom, and the bottom-most square rising to the top left.

51, Set B; **52**, Set A; **53**, neither set; **54**, neither set; **55**, Set A

Explanation

This difficult question has multiple interacting rules.

For Set A, if you see a plus sign, the arrow points right; if you see a minus sign, the arrow points left. Additionally, if you see a circle horizontally next to the plus or minus sign, the arrow is white; if you see no circle in horizontal alignment with the plus or minus sign, the arrow is black.

For Set B, if you see a plus sign, the arrow points left; if you see a minus sign, the arrow points right. Additionally, if you see a circle horizontally next to the plus or minus sign, the arrow is black; if you see no circle in horizontal alignment with the plus or minus sign, the arrow is white.

Test shapes 52 and 55 are Set A, and test shape 51 is Set B. Test shape 53 has the correct arrow direction for Set A but also the correct colour for Set B, and so falls within neither set. Test shape 54 lacks an arrow altogether and so belongs to neither set.

Don't be discouraged if you think that you'll never be able to spot this sort of correlation on test day. This is an example of a seriously hard set of questions that few people can answer correctly.

Chapter 7

Deciphering the Code: The Decision Analysis Subtest

. . . .

In This Chapter

▶ Understanding what the decision analysis subtest looks for

▶ Exploring strategies to answer decision analysis questions quickly

▶ Practising decision analysis questions

. . . .

*T*he decision analysis subtest is all about making judgement calls.

In this subtest, you use a code to unscramble coded phrases into English and to encode English phrases into the code.

At first glance, the concept is straightforward. The catch is that the code lacks the breadth you need to translate fully and explicitly to and from English. The code covers concepts rather than letters, so translation is as much an exercise in manipulating concepts as in looking up items in the code.

Playing around with concepts and manipulating their meaning requires a high level of decision-making ability – which the testers want to check that you have.

Imagine a consultant on call one evening. This consultant deals with GPs who phone to ask the on-call medical team at the hospital to see certain patients. The most junior member of the on-call team on any given day used to do this task, but nowadays more senior members of the team take on the job, because it requires experience and judgement to make decisions.

A GP calls to say that a patient in his surgery has limb weakness. The GP is concerned that the patient may be having a stroke and wants to send him into hospital. The GP has done some initial history-taking and physical examination, but he lacks immediate access to the advanced diagnostic testing and treatments available at the hospital.

The consultant and the GP discuss the patient over the phone. The GP doesn't have all the data to know for sure whether the patient needs hospital treatment. The patient may be having a stroke – but on the other hand, he may have a less urgent complaint.

The consultant prioritises the urgency of the patient's symptoms using the conceptual framework he knows from his training and slotting the limited information the GP has supplied into that framework. Not accepting a seriously ill patient for review would be a serious error, but seeing patients with non-urgent complaints takes time away from more seriously ill patients.

Triaging requires quick decision-making skills. The UKCAT decision analysis subtest checks that you have the innate aptitude to make such decisions.

In this chapter, we explain the types of question found in the decision analysis subtest, suggest useful test strategies and include plenty of practice questions, with answers and fully worked-through explanations.

Decoding the Format of the Decision Analysis Subtest

In this subtest, you have to read a scenario and then answer 28 questions based on the scenario. You have 34 minutes to complete the subtest.

The scenario typically involves a brief paragraph of prose outlining the basic context of the scenario, followed by a table full of data. The questions are based around codes built from the data in the table.

Unlike questions in the other subtests, decision analysis questions have four or five response options, and more than one answer may be correct. The question states whether you need to select more than one answer.

Each of the questions in the decision analysis subtest is in the form of a coded message that you have to decode into English, or an English phrase that you have to encode. The code covers concepts and is not a simple letter-for-letter substitution, so your decisions about which symbols to use and what order to place them in may be ambiguous. You can also combine symbols to alter their meaning, which creates further complexity. Examiners can use commas and parentheses to help organise the symbols into phrases.

For example, suppose that you have a symbol for hot and a symbol for earth. Combining the two symbols may mean hot earth, but you can also use the combination to describe hot sand or even lava. The decision analysis subtest uses this inherent ambiguity to make the questions increasingly complex as the subtest progresses.

You must also select a confidence rating of 1–5 for each of your answers. This is an expression of how sure you are that the answer is right, with 5 being the most confident.

The confidence rating is included only as a trial element of the UKCAT in 2013. Your score on the confidence ratings will not be passed on to universities in 2013. However, the confidence rating is likely to become an official part of the test in future years.

It makes sense to ask about the confidence of your answers. Universities want to know that you can reflect wisely on your limits. Clinicians sometimes face situations where they're not sure of the best way to proceed, and the most appropriate thing to do is to ask for advice. By testing your confidence in your answers, universities check that you are neither over- or under-confident in your decision-making abilities, even while stretching them to their limits.

Being honest about your degree of confidence in your answers is the best way to impress universities with your ability to correctly judge your own performance.

Unlike some of the other subtests in the UKCAT, this subtest rewards lateral thinking and an ability to apply judgement rather than pure logic to situations.

Preparing for Success in the Decision Analysis Subtest

The decision analysis subtest rewards good judgement, which generally comes with experience. Because the subtest is basically a series of puzzles, doing similar puzzles can help you to build up a lot of experience quickly.

Any puzzle that stretches your ability to think and requires lateral thinking can help you with the decision analysis subtest. Riddles are one example, but the most accessible example is newspaper crosswords, especially the cryptic variety. Cryptic crosswords encourage you to think outside the box, drawing on common concepts and conventions which you then apply to the clues. If you already enjoy cryptic crosswords, you'll probably find the decision analysis subtest right up your street.

If you're not a crossword fan, don't worry. Other ways to improve your ability in the decision analysis subtest include creative writing (which encourages the manipulation of ideas and words), simply thinking about how you make real-life decisions (what facts you use, how you combine the facts, and how much weight you give each fact), and practising the questions in this book.

A surprisingly effective way to practise for this subtest is to keep a diary. People constantly think and feel lots of different things, but we rarely take time to understand why we think and feel those things. Developing insight into your emotions and actions requires you to place some sort of logical framework around those fleeting impulses. Doing so means translating – or decoding – emotional states into concepts, and then encoding those concepts into prose. Ordering the concepts into a narrative structure is the essence of good diary-keeping. Try to make your diary a developed explanation of what the day meant to you, rather than random 'blurtings'.

Making the Right Decisions on Test Day

The decision analysis subtest comes at the end of the UKCAT. By the time you get to this subtest, you'll probably already feel tired. Unfortunately, the decision analysis subtest requires you to be at your freshest and sharpest.

Try to clear your mind before you start the decision analysis subtest by using some of these techniques that we recommend:

- **Relax for ten seconds before you start the subtest.** You're under time pressure, but losing ten seconds isn't the end of the world. Those ten seconds of relaxation may be just the ticket to refresh yourself. Take a few deep breaths in and out, focus on slowing your breathing, and try to imagine yourself in a happy and relaxed environment.

- **Don't be intimidated by the large amount of data at the start of the subtest.** You may see lots of unusual symbols, some of which are annoyingly similar to each other. Mentally acknowledge the information and then move on to the test questions.

- **Try to think in concepts, not words.** If you can consider that words and language are merely a human construct applied to underlying concepts, you may find the questions much easier. Your job is to fit a round peg into a square hole – just like in real life when you put your thoughts or feelings into words.

> ✔ **Accept that the questions are deliberately ambiguous.** Feeling some doubt about your answers is normal. Don't spend ages going over a question again and again. Keep moving methodically through the subtest – you have just over one minute per question.
>
> ✔ **Remember that the UKCAT is almost over after you've finished this subtest.** Try to summon the strength to keep going for just a little longer.

The easiest way to understand how these strategies work in practice is to do some questions, see how the answers are derived, and discover how to deal with the complexity and ambiguity of some of the later questions.

Practising Decision Analysis

Working through this section is a good way to practise your decision analysis skills. We include 28 questions in total, just like in the real UKCAT test. Concentrate on thinking in terms of the concepts required by the translation and moving methodically through each question.

Don't be discouraged if you make some mistakes. The whole point of this book is to prepare you for the actual test. Making a few mistakes now means that you're less likely to make the same mistakes on test day.

Avoid rushing through this section. We include full sample tests in Part III for you to do under mock exam conditions. For now, concentrate on understanding the answers and doing the best you can, even if you take a little longer than you have in the real thing. Speed comes with practice and with confidence in the technique.

Scenario

The Symbolians

The Terran Star Navy has a primary mission of seeking out new alien civilisations. On a mission to a previously unexplored planet, it encounters a race without vocal cords. Instead, the alien Symbolians 'speak' using a bioluminescent patch on their faces that is under their conscious control in such a way as to be able to display intricate glowing patterns that form symbols.

First contact with this alien species was difficult, because the Star Navy's Ubiquitous English Device can't translate the pictorial Symbolian language. However, the Star Navy crew has been able to work out some rudimentary translations of symbols through trial and error. The crew's primitive dictionary is shown in Table 7-1.

Table 7-1		The Symbolian Language			
Things		**Descriptors**	**Emotions**	**Times**	
Spaceship = ✈		Enlarge = ▶▶	Angry = ✺	Now = ▶	
Planet = ●		Shrink = ◀◀	Calm = ☙	Later = ▼	
Symbolian = 🕷		Metal = ⅄	Friendly = ♥	Never = ▶▶▌	
Terran = ⚜		Wooden = ♠	Shy = ⊖	Maybe = _	
House = 🏠		Hot = ⓘ			
City = 🏙		Cold = ✛			
Farmland = 🚜					
Road = ▰					
Laser = ∕					
Book = ■					
Ground Car = 🚌					

1. What is the best interpretation of the following Symbolian message?

▶▶ ⚜ ⅄ ✈, ⓘ

A. The large Terran metal spaceship is hot.

B. The large Terran spaceship is made of metal.

C. The large Terran spaceship is cold.

D. The Terran spaceship got hot on landing.

E. The Terran spaceship got larger as it heated up.

2. What is the best interpretation of the following Symbolian message?

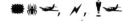

A. The Symbolian spaceship and Terran spaceship fired lasers at each other.

B. The Symbolian spaceship fired at the hostile Terran spaceship.

C. The Terran spaceship fired at the Symbolian spaceship.

D. The Symbolian spaceship fired multiple lasers at the Terran spaceship.

E. The hostile Symbolian spaceship fired lasers at the Terran spaceship.

3. What is the best way to translate the following into Symbolian?

The Terran driving the ground car ruthlessly crashed into the Symbolian.

A. ✹, (✦ ⋯)✸, ❗🚌

B. (✦ ⋯)❗, 🚌✸, ✹

C. ❗🚌, (✦ ⋯)✸, ✹

D. ❗, ✸, ✹

E. (✦ ⋯)🚌, ❗, ✹

4. What is the best interpretation of the following coded message?

❗♥▾, ■, ✹(✹🏠)

A. The Terran will steal the book from the Symbolian's house.

B. The Symbolian angrily took the book back from the Terran.

C. The Terran will give the book as a present to the Symbolian in his home.

D. The Terran spaceship teleports the book into the Symbolian's house.

E. The Terran's house contains a Symbolian book.

5. What is the best interpretation of the following coded message?

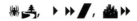

A. Symbolians' farmland is increasingly being converted into roads as their cities expand.

B. Symbolian roads connect farming areas to cities.

C. Symbolian cities are getting smaller as farmland and road networks enlarge.

D. Symbolian farms are so profitable that they support the cities.

E. Farms and cities on Symbolia are both expanding as the road network improves.

6. What is the best interpretation of the following coded message?

❗⟷⟷, ▾✸⁄●, ✹✹⊖, ▸🏠◂◂

A. The spaceship urgently fired lasers at the Symbolian house.

B. The Symbolian base opened fire on the orbiting Terran spaceship.

C. The Symbolians ran out of their house, firing on the Terran spaceship.

D. The Terran Space Navy is threatening orbital bombardment should the Symbolian fugitives not immediately emerge from their hiding place.

E. The Symbolian High Command declared war on the Terran Space Navy.

7. What is the best interpretation of the following coded message?

●①〞, ▾, 🕷⛰🏙, ⫷, ♥

A. As a result of global nuclear war, the Symbolian civilisation collapsed to a pre-technological level of development.
B. Symbolian technology led to global warming.
C. Living on a hot planet, the Symbolians found it easy to develop advanced technology.
D. Symbolian cities went up in flames during their dark ages.
E. As a result of global warming, the Symbolian civilisation collapsed to a pre-technological level of development.

8. What is the best interpretation of the following coded message?

⫷(❗🕷), 〞, (❗)(🕷)

A. Symbolian children are taller than Terran children.
B. Symbolian–Terran hybrid children are taller than either species.
C. Symbolian–Terran hybrid children are shorter than Symbolian children.
D. Symbolians and Terrans cannot interbreed to produce hybrid children.
E. Symbolian–Terran hybrid children are looked down on by both species.

9. What is the best interpretation of the following coded message?

🕷⛏, 〞(🕸①⚱✦)

A. Symbolians poured molten metal over their farmland.
B. Symbolian bridges span deep ravines in their countryside.
C. Symbolians don't like their harsh countryside.
D. Symbolia has many dangerous molten metal rivers outside its cities.
E. Symbolians want to see new planets with exciting farming techniques.

10. What is the best interpretation of the following coded message?

〞(❗✈✈), ⫷(🕷✈✈), ▾〞🕸, ❗●

A. The Symbolian fleet fought the Terran Space Navy over Earth.
B. It took a battle in Earth's orbit for the Terran Space Navy to defeat the Symbolians.
C. The Terran Space Navy engaged the Symbolian fleet over Symbolia.
D. Earth declared war on Symbolia by launching a Space Navy attack.
E. The Symbolian fleet can never defeat Earth, because it's outnumbered by the Terran Space Navy.

11. What is the best interpretation of the following coded message?

⚕🚌🚌, ▼ (▶ ▼)

A. Symbolians never built the roads to support their ground cars.

B. Symbolians never let their ground cars run late.

C. Symbolian ground cars always run late.

D. The Symbolians will catch the later ground car.

E. The ground car will come later to pick up the Symbolians.

12. What is the best interpretation of the following coded message?

⚡⚕❤', – ·· , ✸(⚡🏃⚕🏃)

A. Symbolians and Terrans are working together in an attempt to solve their mutual farming crisis.

B. Symbolians like Terrans because the Terrans solved the Symbolians' farming crisis.

C. Terrans used the Symbolian solution to countryside deforestation, on Earth.

D. Both Earth and Symbolia suffered from a severe food production problem.

E. A joint solution to the Terran–Symbolian farming crisis is impossible.

13. What is the best interpretation of the following coded message?

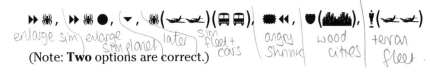

(Note: **Two** options are correct.)

A. 'The primitive Terran Space Navy will be no match for our space and ground forces', the Symbolian admiral cried to rally the planet.

B. The Terran Space Navy has been defeated by the Symbolian Admiral's forces.

C. The Terran Space Navy blockaded Symbolia, causing the Symbolians' leader to charge at them in his spaceship.

D. The Symbolian prime minister intends to attack primitive Earth with his fleet and army.

E. The Symbolian admiral encouraged his people by telling them that the inferior Terran fleet would fall to their fleet and army.

14. What is the best interpretation of the following coded message?

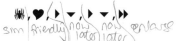

(Note: **Two** options are correct.)

A. The Symbolian loved playing 'Forever and For Always' loudly.

B. The Symbolian currently likes 'It's Now or Never' a lot.

C. The Symbolian enjoys playing 'Never Forget' loudly.

D. The Symbolian loved listening to 'We Have All the Time in the World' many times.

E. The Symbolian listens to 'Time after Time'.

15. What is the best interpretation of the following coded message?

    ❗, ⊖♥, ⚡ ✎ ■, 🕷

    A. The Terran was reluctant to loan the Symbolian his e-book reader.
    B. The Terran secretly liked the Symbolian because of his large library.
    C. The Symbolian had an advanced electronic library of Terran books.
    D. The Terran felt that the Symbolian was hiding e-books from him.
    E. The Symbolian liked the Terran enough to lend him the technical books he wanted.

16. What is the best interpretation of the following coded message?

    ❗● ✈, ⚡(🏭 🏭), ①🚗, ▼, ♥🚗

    A. Terran ships convert desert planets into arable planets.
    B. Terran colony ships contain technology to convert desert into farmland.
    C. Terran colony ships were launched because Earth's farmland was turned into desert.
    D. Large technologically advanced Terran ships seek out new hot arable planets.
    E. The Terran Space Navy uses advanced technology to subjugate both desert and arable planets.

17. What is the best interpretation of the following coded message?

    🕷🏠, _ , ✺✚

    (Note: **Two** options are correct.)

    A. The Symbolian moved home because of changeable weather.
    B. The Symbolian might move home because of the cold weather.
    C. The Symbolian's home planet is often cold.
    D. Symbolian homes are cold and draughty.
    E. The Symbolian's home might be uprooted in a winter storm.

18. What is the best interpretation of the following coded message?

    ❗🚃, _✺, 🕷🚗✈

    A. Terran ground cars are prone to breaking down on Symbolian country roads.
    B. Terran ground cars sometimes drive down Symbolian country roads.
    C. Terran ground cars aren't often found on Symbolian roads.
    D. Terran ground cars are sometimes found on Symbolian roads.
    E. Terrans often avoid using their ground cars on Symbolian country roads.

19. Which **two** of the following would be the most useful additions to our translated knowledge of the Symbolian language when attempting to convey the following message?

    Terran bridges are much more likely to undergo metal fatigue than Symbolian ones, because they are made from inferior metal that undergoes more deformation on extended use.

    A. Deformation

    B. Worse

    C. Fatigue

    D. Bridge

    E. Usage

20. What is the best interpretation of the following coded message?

    !✹, ⊖(▶ ✹ ▼ !■), ✹🚌

    A. The Terran couldn't drive his car, because the instruments were all in Symbolian.

    B. The Symbolian could drive his car on Terran roads, because he understood Terran.

    C. The Terran got frustrated with the lack of a Terran translation for the manual in his Symbolian hire car.

    D. The Terran refused to get into the Symbolian's car.

    E. The Terran laughed at the lack of a Terran translation for the construction manual for his Symbolian kit car.

21. What is the best way to translate the following into Symbolian?

    The wreckage of the ancient Symbolian spaceship was found orbiting one of Symbolia's moons.

    A. ✹(▷▷ ▶ ▷▷ ▼)⤳, ✹●, ✹◀◀

    B. ✹◀◀, ✹(▶ ▼)⤳, ✹●◀◀

    C. ✹◀◀, ✹(_ ▶ _ ▼)⤳, ✹●◀◀

    D. ✹▶▶, ✹(▷▷ ▶ ▷▷ ▼)⤳, ✹●▶▶

    E. ✹◀◀, ✹(▷▷ ▶ ▷▷ ▼)⤳, ✹●◀◀

22. What is the best interpretation of the following coded message?

    !(╱■), ✹▶▶, ●●●

    (Note: **Two** options are correct.)

    A. Terran television is the worst in the galaxy.

    B. Terran telecommunications are the best in the galaxy.

    C. Terrans use electronic communication systems to stay in touch across the galaxy.

    D. Terran email is plagued by spammers in every colony.

    E. The Terrans spent a fortune upgrading their inferior information database.

23. What is the best interpretation of the following coded message?

    ♥, ❗▸▸(🏘️), ♥◂◂, ❗◂◂(🏭▸▸)

    A. I would like to be wealthy enough to buy houses in the country and the city.
    B. I would rather own two houses than a big city.
    C. I would rather be first in a village than second in Rome.
    D. The big Terran liked his two houses in the countryside and his small one in the city.
    E. The Terran bought two big houses and one small city.

24. What is the best way to translate the following into Symbolian?

    This world is the best of all possible worlds.

    A. ●, (●●●)
    B. ●, _, (●●●)
    C. ●, ♥♥(●●●)
    D. ♥▸▸●, (●●●)
    E. ✳▸▸●, ♥(●●●)

25. What is the best interpretation of the following coded message?

    ❗❗, ‥♥, (❗❗)♥

    A. Men like spending time with other men.
    B. Mankind will always like strong leaders.
    C. Men are doomed to be ruled over by tyrants.
    D. The husbands hated their wives.
    E. Men freely believe that which they desire.

26. What is the best interpretation of the following coded message?

    ♥⌖, ✳①, (❗❗)▸▸

    A. The fire on the old galleon caused many deaths.
    B. The sailing ship was brutally hot on deck.
    C. Many people died when cosmic radiation penetrated the spaceship.
    D. The spaceship passed through a solar storm, with few fatalities.
    E. The spaceship passed through the solar storm, but with many fatalities.

27. What is the best interpretation of the following Symbolian message?

    ▸▸,♥,✳, ▸ ,▸▸

    A. Never trust a Symbolian, neither now nor ever.
    B. Symbolians dream of the future.
    C. Never ever love a Symbolian.
    D. Terrans and Symbolians have never been on friendly terms.
    E. Never be friendly with a Symbolian.

28. What is the best interpretation of the following Symbolian message?

    ✳(▸▸⌖)▸▸❗(▸▸⌖)

    A. The Terrans will overpower the Symbolians.
    B. The Terran fleet outnumbers the Symbolian fleet.
    C. The Symbolians will overpower the Terrans.
    D. The Symbolians have faster spaceships than the Terrans have.
    E. The Symbolian fleet outnumbers the Terran fleet.

Answers

1. A: The large Terran metal spaceship is hot.

   ▶▌ ❗ ♨ �, ①

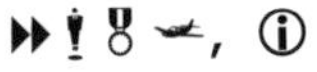

   = Enlarge Terran Metal Spaceship, Hot

   = The large Terran metal spaceship is hot

   The first symbol, 'enlarge', eliminates choice D, because D makes no mention of spaceship size. The other four choices all have 'Terran spaceship', but C and E skip mentioning 'metal'. Between A and B, only B interprets the 'hot' symbol. Note that the comma separates the phrase describing the spaceship from the fact that it became hot.

   You therefore need to pay attention to the literal translation of the symbols, the placement of commas to group ideas or clauses together, and the relationships between these clauses in the sentence being translated. In this first example, doing so is straightforward, but when a large number of symbols and commas are used, the degree of ambiguity in translation rises, forcing you to sometimes decide which option is best, or even 'least worst'. This inherent ambiguity is a deliberate part of the test.

2. E: The hostile Symbolian spaceship fired lasers at the Terran spaceship.

   ✺ 👾 ⚓, ✎, ❗⚓

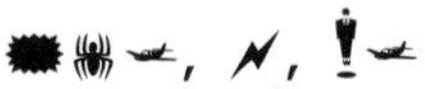

3. B: (✚ ••)❗, 🚌 ✺, 👾

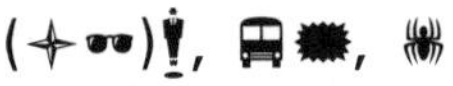

   The Terran driving the ground car ruthlessly crashed into the Symbolian.

   = Angry Symbolian Spaceship, Laser, Terran Spaceship

   = The hostile Symbolian spaceship fired lasers at the Terran spaceship

   = (✚ ••)❗, 🚌 ✺, 👾

   = Ruthless Terran, Ground Car Hostile, Symbolian

   = (Cold Calm) Terran, Ground Car Angry, Symbolian

4. C: The Terran will give the book as a present to the Symbolian in his home.

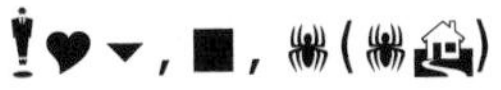

   ❗♥ ▼, ■, 👾 (👾 🏠)

= Terran Friendly Later, Book, Symbolian (Symbolian Home)

= The Terran will be friendly, book, Symbolian in his home

= The Terran will do something friendly with the book to the Symbolian in his home

= The Terran will give the book as a present to the Symbolian in his home

The first three symbols tell us 'Terran friendly later', which refers to the Terran being friendly in the future. Choice A says that the Terran is unfriendly in the future, and choice B makes no mention of the Terran being friendly later, but instead says that the Terran is angry now. The last three symbols translate to Symbolian (Symbolian home). E incorrectly translates this phrase to 'the Terran home'. D doesn't refer to the Symbolian playing a part in the transaction. This brings us to C.

5. A: Symbolians' farmland is increasingly being converted into roads as their cities expand.

= Symbolian Farmland, Now Enlarge Road, City Enlarge

= Symbolian farmland, now more roads, cities expand

= Symbolian farmland is increasingly being converted into roads as their cities expand

B contains no information about the changes in size. C applies the wrong changes in size, as does E. D talks about profitability, which isn't included in the code, and doesn't mention the roads.

6. D: The Terran Space Navy is threatening orbital bombardment should the Symbolian fugitives not immediately emerge from their hiding place.

= Terran Spaceship Spaceship, Later Angry Laser Planet, Symbolian Symbolian Shy, Now House Shrink

= Terran Space Navy, will fire lasers on planet, Symbolians shy now shrink from house

= The Terran Space Navy will fire lasers on planet if the Symbolian fugitives don't right now leave their house

= The Terran Space Navy is threatening orbital bombardment should the Symbolian fugitives not immediately emerge from their hiding place

7. E: As a result of global warming, the Symbolian civilisation collapsed to a pre-technological level of development.

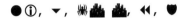

= Planet Hot, Later, Symbolian City City, Shrink, Wooden

= Planet warming, caused Symbolian cities, shrink to wooden

= Global warming caused Symbolian civilisation to collapse to wooden

= As a result of global warming, the Symbolian civilisation collapsed to a pre-technological level of development

The question uses the word 'wooden' to describe a more primitive technology. To decipher this question, you need to accept that because wooden things generally precede metal things, then if the Symbolian city (civilisation) is now wooden, and it got here by shrinking, the earlier civilisation must have been more technologically advanced.

This need to apply lateral thinking illustrates a difference between this subtest and the verbal reasoning subtest. The verbal reasoning subtest requires you to use only simple logic, but decision analysis allows and requires you to manipulate concepts and merge them together.

8. B: Symbolian–Terran hybrid children are taller than either species.

◀◀ (⟱ ⟱), ▶▶, (⟱) (⟱)

= Shrink (Terran Symbolian), Enlarge, (Terran)(Symbolian)

= Small (product of Terran and Symbolian), bigger, (Terran) (Symbolian)

= Terran–Symbolian hybrid children are bigger than Terrans and Symbolians

= Terran–Symbolian hybrid children are taller than either species

Note that the question uses the same set of symbols (those for 'enlarge' and 'shrink') to conduct two different operations within the same code, based on placement of parentheses. This is an example of why you need imagination and lateral thinking when you encode or decode using a restricted set of symbols. The translation is a little uncertain, but you can still find a best interpretation. In question 10, 'shrink' is used as a description, whereas here it's used as an operation. If used descriptively in this case, it can be translated as 'Hybrid is small; Terran and Symbolian both large', which is the opposite of the desired meaning.

9. D: Symbolia has many dangerous molten metal rivers outside its cities.

 # 🛋, ▶(✹①♋/)

= Symbolian Farmland, Enlarge(Angry Hot Metal Road)

= Symbolian farmland has many angry molten metal roads

= Symbolian countryside has many dangerous molten metal rivers

= Symbolian has many dangerous molten metal rivers outside its cities

10. E: The Symbolian fleet can never defeat Earth, because it's outnumbered by the Terran Space Navy.

▶(❗⤴⤴), ◀(✹⤴⤴), ▼ ▶✹, ❗●

= Enlarge (Terran Spaceship Spaceship), Shrink (Symbolian Spaceship Spaceship), Later Never Angry, Terran Planet

= Large Terran fleet small Symbolian fleet could never angry Earth

= The Terran fleet outnumbers the Symbolian fleet could never defeat Earth

= The Symbolian fleet could never defeat Earth, because it's outnumbered by the Terran Space Navy

11. C: Symbolian ground cars always run late.

#🚌🚌, ▼(▶▼)

= Symbolian Ground Car Ground Car, Later (Now Later)

= Symbolian ground cars, later (always)

= Symbolian ground cars are always later

= Symbolian ground cars always run late

12. A: Symbolians and Terrans are working together in an attempt to solve their mutual farming crisis.

❗#♥, –⚬⚬, ✹(❗🛋#🛋)

= Terran Symbolian Friendly, Maybe Calm, Angry (Terran Farmland Symbolian Farmland)

= Terrans and Symbolians friendly to maybe calm, angry (mutual farmland)

= Terrans and Symbolians are working together to possibly calm the mutual farmland crisis

= Symbolians and Terrans are working together in an attempt to solve the their mutual farming crisis

13. A: 'The primitive Terran Space Navy will be no match for our space and ground forces', the Symbolian admiral cried to rally the planet.

And

E: The Symbolian admiral encouraged his people by telling them that the inferior Terran Fleet would fall to their fleet and army.

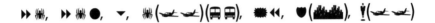

= Enlarge Symbolian, Enlarge Symbolian Planet, Later, Symbolian (Spaceship Spaceship) (Ground Car Ground Car), Angry Shrink, Wooden (City City), Terran (Spaceship Spaceship)

= Major Symbolian, make all Symbolian people bigger, later, Symbolian fleet and Symbolian ground troops, aggressively shrink, primitive civilisation, Terran fleet

= The Symbolian admiral encouraged his people that later Symbolian fleet and army defeat primitive Terran fleet

= 'The primitive Terran Space Navy will be no match for our space and ground forces', the Symbolian admiral cried to rally the planet

And

= The Symbolian admiral encouraged his people by telling them that the inferior Terran fleet would fall to their fleet and army

English is a versatile language, and often you can use many phrases to give the same essential meaning. If you parse down the sentences in this question into their basic meanings, you can see that answers A and E say the same thing. The kind of conceptual code that the Symbolians use (and, indeed, that you find in the decision analysis subtest in general) is much stricter than English, because the code has fewer ways of expressing any given idea.

A quick way to solve questions where more than one answer is correct is to look for pairs of equivalent but differently phrased answers. If you can see only one pair of answers in the set of options and the question asks you to choose two options, that pair of answers is probably correct.

Be careful not to get caught out using this shortcut in questions that contain two pairs of equivalent options.

14. A: The Symbolian loved playing 'Forever and For Always' loudly.

And

D: The Symbolian loved listening to 'We Have All the Time in the World' many times.

⧉ , ♥ , ▶ ▼ , ▶ ▼ , ▶▶

= Symbolian, Friendly, Now Later, Now Later, Enlarge

= The Symbolian loves forever always loudly/many

= The Symbolian loved playing 'Forever and For Always' loudly

And

= The Symbolian loved listening to 'We Have All the Time in the World' many times

This question creates the rather odd mental image of an alien getting down to Shania Twain and Louis Armstrong. The question is also a more subtle exploration of the ambiguity you may find in the decision analysis subtest. Some elements of the answers don't exist in the code, forcing you to fill in the gaps in small ways. For example, no code exists for 'playing' or 'listening'.

This makes excluding the other answer options harder. You can rule out B, because the middle two pairs of symbols are the same, not opposites. You can also exclude C: adding in elements to account for 'never', 'forget' and 'playing' is more of a manipulation of the code's translation than the two correct answers, which involve the addition of a maximum of two elements. Finally, E doesn't fully express the 'friendly' symbol, so isn't the best interpretation.

A is the better of the two remaining interpretations, as 'forever' is synonymous with 'for always'. D is a harder conceptual stretch, and if the question only asked for a single answer, could be excluded. However, the question asks for two answers, and D is the second best translation.

15. A: The Terran was reluctant to loan the Symbolian his e-book reader.

⚡ , ⊖♥ , ⚇ ⟋ ■ , ⧉

= Terran, Shy Friendly, Metal Laser Book, Symbolian

= The Terran, reluctant be nice, e-book reader, to Symbolian

= The Terran was reluctant to loan the Symbolian his e-book reader

C, D and E can all be excluded on the basis of the subject and object of the sentence not matching the order of the code.

Neither A nor B are ideal translations, so you must choose the least worst. A is superior, because translating 'shy friendly' into 'reluctant' is less hard than translating 'metal laser book' into 'large library'. Choosing between two frustratingly but not equally poor options sometimes happens in this subtest.

Being open to the potential alternative and metaphorical meanings of unusual collections of symbols, but still being alert to maintaining the syntactical meaning of the code, is challenging. You need to be imaginative and to work within boundaries at the same time.

 In any real-life decision-making situation, hard decisions are hard precisely because you can neither ignore the limits of reality nor use conventional solutions to solve the problem. Harnessing your imagination is the key to good decision-making.

16. B: Terran colony ships contain technology to convert desert into farmland.

    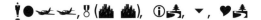

    = Terran Planet Spaceship Spaceship, Metal (City City), Hot Farmland, Later, Friendly Farmland

    = Terran planet ships, advanced civilisation, desert, later, farmland

    = Terran colony ships have technology desert become farmland

    = Terran colony ships contain technology to convert desert into farmland

    In this question, the 'friendly' symbol next to the second 'farmland' symbol acts as a contextual contrast to the 'hot' symbol next to the first 'farmland' symbol. If you later convert 'hot farmland' to 'friendly farmland', you can deduce that the original hotness wasn't the friendly hotness associated with lots of sunshine over fertile land, but was the unfriendly hotness of a desert.

17. B: The Symbolian might move home because of the cold weather.

    And

    E: The Symbolian's home might be uprooted in a winter storm.

    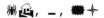

    = Symbolian House, Maybe, Angry Cold

    = The Symbolian house may cold is bad

    = The Symbolian might move home because of the cold weather

And

= The Symbolian's home might be uprooted in a winter storm

Although no code exists for 'moving' or 'uprooting', only these two options include all the other translations of the symbols used in the question, retain their relationships to each other, and introduce the fewest additional elements.

18. A: Terran ground cars are prone to breaking down on Symbolian country roads.

!◫, _❋, ▥⛟/

= Terran Ground Car, Maybe Angry, Symbolian Farmland Road

= Terran ground cars, can become angry, Symbolian country roads

= Terran grounds cars are prone to breaking down on Symbolian country roads

Neither the code for 'ground car' nor the code for 'road' is repeated to indicate plurality in the Symbolian message, unlike usage in previous questions. However, as all the potential answer options use plural forms, no extra ambiguity results. If the meaning is clear, sometimes Symbolians don't bothering pluralising.

English has its fair share of variable and sloppy usage but still retains contextual meaning. If you use abbreviations when you text your friends, you're probably guilty of significantly worse omissions.

19. A: Deformation

And

D: Bridge

This question is quite difficult. All the possible answers would help to convey the message. In addition, you can send the message by combining existing symbols in the Symbolian language. The question asks you to decide which extra terms would be most helpful – in other words, which new symbols give you the most bang for your buck in conveying the message.

Choosing 'bridge' as one answer is relatively straightforward. Conveying the full meaning of a bridge using the existing symbols is quite difficult. Combining 'metal' and 'road' gives you some sense of what a bridge is but lacks the concept of it being *above* something. As a last resort, you can try to use the 'enlarge' symbol to convey the bridge being above something, but this option is unsatisfactory, as the 'enlarge' symbol would more logically mean 'bigger' rather than 'above'.

Choosing 'deformation' as the other correct answer is a bit harder. You can depict the concept of deformation fairly accurately using the Symbolian equivalent of something along the lines of 'Now, Later, Now Maybe, Later Maybe'. But this expression is quite a mouthful – or should we say 'eyeful' in the case of the Symbolian language!

You can convey the options of 'worse', 'fatigue' and 'usage' more simply using the existing symbols. 'Worse' can be 'Enlarge Angry'. 'Fatigue' can be 'Angry', because you need to convey the stress associated with metal fatigue rather than a sense of sleepiness. You can omit 'usage' altogether from the message, because the other elements of the message imply this concept.

Adding a symbol for 'deformation' alongside one for 'bridge' is more efficient than any of the other options.

20. C: The Terran got frustrated with the lack of a Terran translation for the manual in his Symbolian hire car.

‼️☀️, ⊖ (▸ 🕷 ▾ ‼️◼️), 🕷 🚌

= Terran Angry, Shy (Now Symbolian Later Terran Book), Symbolian Ground Car

= Terran angry, shy (Terran translation book), Symbolian car

= Terran angry, lack of (Terran translation book), Symbolian car

= The Terran got frustrated with the lack of a Terran translation for the manual in his Symbolian hire car

21. E: ☀️◀◀, 🕷 (⏭ ▸ ⏭ ▾)↩︎, 🕷 ⬤ ◀◀

= Angry Shrink, Symbolian (Never Now Never Later) Spaceship, Symbolian Planet Shrink

= Break into smaller bits, Symbolian (not present nor future) spaceship, Symbolian smaller than planet

= Wrecked, Symbolian (past) spaceship, Symbolian moon

= The wreckage of the ancient Symbolian spaceship was found orbiting one of Symbolia's moons

22. A: Terran television is the worst in the galaxy.

And

D: Terran email is plagued by spammers in every colony.

‼️(✎ ◼️), ☀️▸▸, ⬤⬤⬤

= Terran (Laser Book), Angry Enlarge, Planet Planet Planet

= Terran television very bad every planet

= Terran television is the worst in the galaxy

And

= Terran (Laser Book), Angry Enlarge, Planet Planet Planet

= Terran email, lots of bad, every planet

= Terran email is plagued by spammers in every colony

23. C: I would rather be first in a village than second in Rome.

♥, ❗▸▸(🏘️🏘️), ♥◂◂, ❗◂◂(🏭▸▸)

= Friendly, Terran Enlarge (House House), Friendly Shrink, Terran Shrink (City Enlarge)

= Like, Terran big (village), like less, Terran small (big city)

= Like first in village, less like second in big city

= I would rather be first in a village than second in Rome

24. D: ♥▸▸●, (●●●)

= Friendly Enlarge Planet, (Planet Planet Planet)

= Like lot planet, all planets

= This world is the best of all possible worlds

Satisfaction

The translation 'I would rather be first in a village than second in Rome' is a paraphrasing of a quote by the ancient philosopher Epicurus, who espoused the value of being happy about being in control of your own life rather than constantly trying to chase greater things. The original quote invoked an Iberian village, but trying to encode Iberian in Symbolian seemed like too much of a big task, even for this question-setter.

A Panglossian outlook

The German philosopher Leibniz first coined the phrase 'This world is the best of all possible worlds' in an attempt to explain why a benevolent and omnipotent god would create a world with such suffering as ours. Leibniz argued that if this world is the one God chose for us, then this world must be the best of all possible worlds that can exist, meaning that all the other possible worlds are even worse. This position was satirised by the French writer Voltaire in *Candide*. Candide's tutor, Dr Pangloss, uses the phrase to raise his spirits when he faces awful personal hardship. This kind of unrelenting and unrealistic optimism is now often termed 'Panglossian'.

25. E: Men freely believe that which they desire.

‼, ⚫⚫♥, (‼)♥

= Terran Terran, Calm Friendly, (Terran Terran) Friendly

= Men, calmly like, what men like

= Men freely believe that which they desire

B, C and D can rapidly be excluded due to those translations including terms absent from the code. It can be argued that A is a valid translation:

Man man, calm friendly, (man man) friendly = Men, subdued happiness, men, happy = Men like spending time with other men. However, this phrase can be translated from Symbolian without the need for the final 'happy' symbol. Its presence indicates an additional layer of meaning, making E the preferable answer, because it makes use of all the components of the code.

Classical psychology

The phrase 'Men freely believe that which they desire' comes from Julius Caesar, Emperor of Rome. This shrewd psychological insight reveals Caesar's innate political talent. The idea is that people are more easily persuaded by a weak argument that focuses on what they want and believe, than by a stronger argument that focuses on what is true. Also, when they make decisions, people generally believe themselves to be motivated by what is right, but other people to be motivated by selfish personal interest. The field of social psychology describes this phenomenon more formally as the 'fundamental attribution error'.

26. A: The fire on the old galleon caused many deaths.

    ♥ ✈, ✺ ①, (❗❗)▸▸|

    = Wooden Spaceship, Angry Hot, (Terran Terran) Never

    = Wooden ship, bad hot, (many people) never

    = Old ship, fire, many died

    = The fire on the old galleon caused many deaths

27. A: Never trust a Symbolian, neither now nor ever.

    ▸▸|, ♥, ✺, ▸, ▸▸|

    = Never, Friendly, Symbolian, Now, Never

    Friendly is being used to convey a sense of mutual trust, so:

    = Never trust a Symbolian, neither now nor ever

28. E: The Symbolian fleet outnumbers the Terran fleet.

    ✺ (▸▸ ✈) ▸▸ ❗ (▸▸ ✈)

    = Symbolian (Enlarge Spaceship), Enlarge, Terran (Enlarge Spaceship)

    'Enlarge Spaceship' becomes 'fleet', with enlarge as a separate term conveying outnumbering, so:

    = The Symbolian fleet outnumbers the Terran fleet.

Chapter 8

Making the Call: The Situational Judgement Subtest

*S*ituational judgement is about making the right choice under tough circumstances. It's the ability to quickly analyse a complex ethical situation, taking into account a variety of competing moral principles, and make a sensible decision about what to do to resolve matters.

The UKCAT tests this skill because health professionals are frequently placed in sensitive situations, and medical and dental schools need to be confident that their students can approach such situations wisely. Medical and dental schools don't expect applicants like you to have all the professional knowledge that a qualified doctor or dentist has. And they don't expect you to be aware of all the detailed ethical advice and guidance that exists to help qualified professionals make the right decision. But they do want to see that you have a basic moral compass and an awareness of complex interacting pressures, and that you have an aptitude for balancing these competing nuances when deciding what to do.

In this chapter, we give you the facts, strategies and practice that you need to do well in the UKCAT situational judgement subtest. We include a detailed explanation of the format of the situational judgement subtest and the types of question you'll face, some useful strategies for developing your ability to identify competing moral principles, essential tips for test day, and plenty of practice scenarios with questions and answers in the form of fully worked-through explanations.

Figuring out the Format of the Situational Judgement Subtest

The situational judgement subtest consists of 17 scenarios. Each scenario is a brief description of a real-world situation that highlights an ethical dilemma.

The scenarios are typically designed to include multiple competing moral principles, so the right way to solve the problem is not always immediately obvious. This ambiguity is a deliberate component of the test: there will often be more than one reasonably correct way to act, as well as a number of incorrect ways.

There are 71 items, or questions, spread across the 17 scenarios, with between 3 and 6 items per scenario. You have 27 minutes to complete the situational judgement subtest.

There are two main types of question:

✔ In the first type, you are asked to assess the *appropriateness* of a range of different responses to the scenario.

✔ In the second type, you have to judge the *importance* of a range of different actions or principles in resolving the scenario.

Each type of question presents its own challenges. To answer the questions it's crucial to understand exactly what the UKCAT examiners mean by each type of question.

UKCAT's definitions of *appropriateness* and *importance* vary slightly from what you might intuitively understand the words to mean. You must use UKCAT's definitions when answering each item.

For the appropriateness questions, UKCAT uses the following definitions to describe the various levels of appropriateness:

✔ **A very appropriate thing to do** will address at least one aspect (not necessarily all aspects) of the situation.

✔ **Appropriate, but not ideal** means it could be done, but is not necessarily a very good thing to do.

✔ **Inappropriate, but not awful** means it should not really be done, but would not be terrible.

✔ **A very inappropriate thing to do** should definitely not be done and would make the situation worse.

Candidates often find it difficult to decide between the various responses, because several steps are needed to resolve a tricky ethical situation.

Don't judge a response as if it's the only thing that is done. In other words, remember that each step may be only part of your overall ideal approach to the problem. Judge each response on its own merits. If it's something you should do, it's going to be appropriate, even if it's not the only thing you do.

For the second type of question, you rate the importance of a series of options in response to the scenario. UKCAT uses the following definitions to decide importance:

- ✔ **Very important** is something that is vital to take into account.

- ✔ **Important** is something that is important but not vital to take into account.

- ✔ **Of minor importance** is something that could be taken into account, but that doesn't really matter.

- ✔ **Not important at all** is something that should definitely not be taken into account.

There is a subtle difference between the appropriateness and importance questions. In the appropriateness questions, the approximate midpoint broadly dividing a 'good thing' from a 'bad thing' is between *appropriate but not ideal* and *inappropriate but not awful*. For the importance questions, the midpoint is between *of minor importance* and *not important at all*.

In other words, within the definitions of the UKCAT, you're given more ways to consider whether something is important than whether something is appropriate. Keeping in mind this broad difference between the two types of question can help you decide whether responses are broadly good things to do or not.

Preparing for Success in the Situational Judgement Subtest

The best way to prepare for this test is to practise thinking about the ethics of any given situation. The whole basis of the test is about being able to quickly spot the nature of the underlying ethical conflict and then decide what needs to be done.

You can practise this kind of thinking in two main ways, and it's worth using both methods:

- ✔ **Do lots of situational judgement questions.** We include plenty of situational judgement questions in this book. Doing lots of questions and reading the answers and explanations carefully gives you exposure to a large range of different scenarios. That means you learn to spot any similar issues in fresh scenarios.

- ✔ **Learn about some key ethical principles.** Then you will have a core framework for approaching any new situation. In this section we highlight some of those principles.

You can further your knowledge by reading around this topic. Sources of information include guidance from the General Medical Council (GMC) on what a doctor should be like. This document, called *Good Medical Practice,* can be found at www.gmc-uk.org/guidance/good_medical_practice.asp. Another good source of information is the book *Medical Ethics: A Very Short Introduction,* by Tony Hope.

Learning some key principles

The care of your patient should always be your first concern; when you're at work, your first duty is helping your patients. Whatever you do needs to be guided by this broad principle of *beneficence.*

You should always work within the limits of your own competence; this means knowing what your limits are, and not doing things you aren't trained for or aren't capable of doing. Obviously, doctors and dentists need to learn how to do things, and sometimes you practise these techniques on patients. But that's done under the supervision of someone who is more fully trained in those techniques. If you're placed in a situation where you feel forced to act outside your limits, you need to be able to seek the help of others who know better. In other words, you should avoid doing harm: *non-maleficence.*

You have to respect patients' dignity, including their right to *confidentiality.* Health professionals have a duty not to share confidential medical information with those outside the patient's care team. A small number of very specific exceptions to this general rule exist, but confidentiality should only be broken with a great deal of forethought.

Patients have a right to make their own choices about their healthcare; this is *autonomy.* Your responsibility is ensuring they have, and understand, all the facts they need to make that decision. In a small number of situations you might have to act without knowing a patient's choice. For example, someone who arrives unconscious in an emergency department and needs life-saving treatment doesn't have the legal capacity to make a choice, and the doctor is obliged to provide treatment anyway. In some situations a health professional can enforce certain types of treatment, such as psychiatric care, but for the situational judgement subtest you're not expected to have that sort of specialist medical or procedural knowledge.

You should always be honest, and never discriminate unfairly. *Justice* is about treating everyone as fairly as possible and in accordance with what your professional guidance says is right.

Philosophically minded candidates will probably enjoy reading further around these issues. The more you understand about how people think and how they decide what's right and wrong, the easier you'll find the situational judgement subtest. However, it's equally important to avoid overcomplicating problems.

You have to place your decisions within the broadly accepted ethical framework used by health professionals and wider society. You might have a complex philosophical justification for choosing an answer other than the 'right' one, but the UKCAT examiners (and medical schools) are looking for people they can train to work within the ethical framework of the health service. That doesn't mean you're not allowed freedom of expression, but you must be willing to make decisions within the protocols and principles of what doctors and dentists generally accept to be true.

Doing well in the situational judgement subtest involves putting yourself in the shoes of a doctor (or examiner) and choosing your answers accordingly.

Using your best judgement on test day

The situational judgement subtest is at the end of the UKCAT, and most people are feeling exhausted by this stage. While it is arguably less mentally taxing that the first four subtests, you still need to think clearly and carefully about your answers.

The following tips will help you score well on test day:

⮞ **Don't get bogged down overthinking a problem.** It's easy to start second-guessing yourself in the situational judgement subtest. Usually, your first instinct is likely to be correct, especially once you've done enough practice to be familiar with the key principles around which many scenarios revolve.

✔ **Bear in mind that the UKCAT examiners understand that there isn't always an absolutely right answer.** They know that ethical problems often include uncertain shades of grey. To address this, you get partial credit for selecting an answer option only one away from what the examiners picked. For example, if the examiners think that the best answer is 'appropriate but not ideal', you'll still get some credit for 'inappropriate, but not awful'. And unlike in the other subtests, your score for this section is given as a band (similar to a grade), with Band 1 being the best and Band 4 the worst. Knowing that you can still be in Band 1 despite answering some questions wrongly should help to reassure you during the test and thereby prevent you from second-guessing yourself.

✔ **Consider each response independently from the other responses.** Don't let your answer to one question affect how you answer a subsequent question. The situational judgement subtest is designed such that each answer can and should be considered in isolation.

✔ **Read the question carefully.** In particular, understand whether it's an appropriateness or importance question, and whose shoes (for example, medical student, doctor, patient or friend) you are asked to put yourself in when deciding between the options.

✔ **Answer all the questions.** Negative marking isn't used, so don't be afraid to guess if you're not sure. You're quite likely to get at least some partial credit if you are close to the right answer.

To see how these tips work in practice, try the questions in the rest of this chapter.

Practising Situational Judgement

In this section, you'll get 71 items associated with 17 scenarios, just like in the UKCAT. The best way to use this section is to read each scenario and then attempt to work out the answers for yourself. We include worked-through answers at the end of the chapter, but try to avoid looking at the answers until you've come up with your own set.

Don't be discouraged if you make mistakes. The whole point of this book is to prepare you for the actual test. Making a few mistakes now means that you're less likely to make the same mistakes on test day.

Avoid rushing through this section. We include full sample tests for you to do under mock exam conditions in Part III. For now, concentrate on understanding the answers and doing the best you can, even if you take a little more time than you will have during the real test. Speed comes with practice and with confidence in the technique.

Your clinical partner can't attend a biochemistry lecture later this afternoon, as she has an appointment at the dentist's. She has asked you to sign the attendance register in her name, because students must attend 90 per cent of lectures if they are to be admitted to the end-of-year exam.

How **appropriate** are each of the following responses by **you** in this situation?

1. Sign the register in your clinical partner's name, because a dental appointment is a valid reason for missing a lecture.

   A. A very appropriate thing to do.
   B. Appropriate, but not ideal.
   C. Inappropriate, but not awful.
   D. A very inappropriate thing to do.

2. Sign the register in your clinical partner's name so that, in the future, she might do the same for you.

   A. A very appropriate thing to do.
   B. Appropriate, but not ideal.
   C. Inappropriate, but not awful.
   D. A very inappropriate thing to do.

3. Sign the register in your clinical partner's name on the grounds that the medical school's rules are petty and ridiculous.

   A. A very appropriate thing to do.
   B. Appropriate, but not ideal.
   C. Inappropriate, but not awful.
   D. A very inappropriate thing to do.

4. Refuse to sign the register in your clinical partner's name, underlining that this would be unethical.

   A. A very appropriate thing to do.
   B. Appropriate, but not ideal.
   C. Inappropriate, but not awful.
   D. A very inappropriate thing to do.

5. Discuss the ethics and possible consequences of falsifying a signature with your clinical partner, and help her explore alternative solutions.

   A. A very appropriate thing to do.
   B. Appropriate, but not ideal.
   C. Inappropriate, but not awful.
   D. A very inappropriate thing to do.

6. Refuse to sign the register in your clinical partner's name and bring up the matter with the academic tutor.

   A. A very appropriate thing to do.
   B. Appropriate, but not ideal.
   C. Inappropriate, but not awful.
   D. A very inappropriate thing to do.

You are a medical student interviewing a patient, when she discloses that she drinks two bottles of wine a day. She tells you not to tell the consultant, but you remember that alcohol can interact with the medication she is taking. You mention this to her, but she insists that you keep quiet about her drinking.

How **important** to take into account are the following considerations for **you** when deciding how to respond to the situation?

7. The patient's right to confidentiality.

    A. Very important.
    B. Important.
    C. Of minor importance.
    D. Not important at all.

8. Whether the patient is actually taking her medication.

    A. Very important.
    B. Important.
    C. Of minor importance.
    D. Not important at all.

9. The nature and possible consequences of the interaction between alcohol and the patient's medication.

    A. Very important.
    B. Important.
    C. Of minor importance.
    D. Not important at all.

10. The patient's opinion of the consultant.

    A. Very important.
    B. Important.
    C. Of minor importance.
    D. Not important at all.

After having had a few beers, your flatmate tells you that his sister, who is studying at another medical school, once wrote an essay for her course in ethics which he recently dug out and submitted as his own work.

How **appropriate** are each of the following responses by **you** in this situation?

11. Discuss the issue with the ethics lecturer at the earliest opportunity.

    A. A very appropriate thing to do.
    B. Appropriate, but not ideal.
    C. Inappropriate, but not awful.
    D. A very inappropriate thing to do.

12. Discuss the issue with your flatmate on the following day, when he is sober.

    A. A very appropriate thing to do.
    B. Appropriate, but not ideal.
    C. Inappropriate, but not awful.
    D. A very inappropriate thing to do.

13. Do nothing and let it pass, because your flatmate was drunk at the time.

    A. A very appropriate thing to do.
    B. Appropriate, but not ideal.
    C. Inappropriate, but not awful.
    D. A very inappropriate thing to do.

14. Do nothing and let it pass, because it's none of your business.

    A. A very appropriate thing to do.
    B. Appropriate, but not ideal.
    C. Inappropriate, but not awful.
    D. A very inappropriate thing to do.

You are a medical student on attachment to a surgical team. One morning, John, the foundation doctor, arrives more than one hour late, and you are sure that you can smell alcohol on his breath. You are friendly with John, and know that he has recently split up with his long-term girlfriend.

How **important** to take into account are the following considerations for **you** when deciding how to respond to the situation?

15. The tasks that John is due to perform on that day.

A. Very important.
B. Important.
C. Of minor importance.
D. Not important at all.

16. John's reputation and career progression.

A. Very important.
B. Important.
C. Of minor importance.
D. Not important at all.

17. The safety of John's patients.

A. Very important.
B. Important.
C. Of minor importance.
D. Not important at all.

18. John's welfare.

A. Very important.
B. Important.
C. Of minor importance.
D. Not important at all.

19. Attenuating circumstances, such as the split-up with the girlfriend.

A. Very important.
B. Important.
C. Of minor importance.
D. Not important at all.

Mrs Dickinson, an in-patient who you have spent a lot of time talking to, is about to be discharged. You come to say goodbye to her, when she hands you an envelope containing a thank-you card together with £100 in cash. When you try to return the money, she refuses to take it back and insists that you deserve to keep it.

How **appropriate** are each of the following responses by **you** in this situation?

20. Explore Mrs Dickinson's motivations for giving you the money.

   A. A very appropriate thing to do.
   B. Appropriate, but not ideal.
   C. Inappropriate, but not awful.
   D. A very inappropriate thing to do.

21. Refuse the money, and ask Mrs Dickinson to buy you something instead.

   A. A very appropriate thing to do.
   B. Appropriate, but not ideal.
   C. Inappropriate, but not awful.
   D. A very inappropriate thing to do.

22. Accept the money, but inform Mrs Dickinson that you will be donating the entire sum to your favourite charity.

   A. A very appropriate thing to do.
   B. Appropriate, but not ideal.
   C. Inappropriate, but not awful.
   D. A very inappropriate thing to do.

23. Tell Mrs Dickinson that accepting a monetary gift is probably against hospital or professional guidelines.

   A. A very appropriate thing to do.
   B. Appropriate, but not ideal.
   C. Inappropriate, but not awful.
   D. A very inappropriate thing to do.

Mrs Jones is very protective of her first child, Noah. When their GP, Dr Aldred, suggests that Noah ought to be vaccinated against mumps, measles and rubella (MMR), Mrs Jones strongly objects.

How **important** to take into account are the following considerations for **Dr Aldred** when deciding how to respond to the situation?

24. Mrs Jones's concerns about the vaccine.

   A. Very important.

   B. Important.

   C. Of minor importance.

   D. Not important at all.

25. The potential risks, both to Noah and to other children, if Noah doesn't receive the vaccine.

   A. Very important

   B. Important.

   C. Of minor importance.

   D. Not important at all.

26. Current guidelines on the administration of the vaccine.

   A. Very important

   B. Important.

   C. Of minor importance.

   D. Not important at all.

27. Financial incentives for delivering vaccinations.

   A. Very important

   B. Important.

   C. Of minor importance.

   D. Not important at all.

28. Mrs Jones's right to refuse the vaccine on behalf of Noah.

   A. Very important.

   B. Important.

   C. Of minor importance.

   D. Not important at all.

Ella, a final-year medical student, is at a cocktail bar with a mixed group of medical and non-medical students when she sees a former patient who was under her care at the same bar. He spots her, comes over and starts talking to her in front of her friends, and asks her out. Ella is attracted to him.

How **appropriate** are each of the following responses by **Ella** in this situation?

29. Pursue a relationship with him, because he's no longer under her care.

    A. A very appropriate thing to do.
    B. Appropriate, but not ideal.
    C. Inappropriate, but not awful.
    D. A very inappropriate thing to do.

30. Tell him that she can't go out with him, because he was a patient in hospital under her care.

    A. A very appropriate thing to do.
    B. Appropriate, but not ideal.
    C. Inappropriate, but not awful.
    D. A very inappropriate thing to do.

31. Decline politely, pretending she's not interested in him in that way.

    A. A very appropriate thing to do.
    B. Appropriate, but not ideal.
    C. Inappropriate, but not awful.
    D. A very inappropriate thing to do.

You are a second-year medical student leaving work. Manoeuvring out of the staff car park, you reverse into a parked car. You recognise the car as belonging to one of the hospital consultants. The bodywork of his car is only slightly dented. There aren't any CCTV cameras and no-one is in the vicinity of the car park.

How **appropriate** are each of the following responses by **you** in this situation?

32. Leave a note, apologising for the mistake and including your insurance details.

A. A very appropriate thing to do.
B. Appropriate, but not ideal.
C. Inappropriate, but not awful.
D. A very inappropriate thing to do.

33. Leave a note apologising for the mistake, omitting contact details because the consultant can afford to repair the car, whereas you can't afford a rise in your insurance premium from a claim.

A. A very appropriate thing to do.
B. Appropriate, but not ideal.
C. Inappropriate, but not awful.
D. A very inappropriate thing to do.

34. Leave a note apologising for the mistake, including your contact details. When you see the consultant, explain the situation to him and ask whether you can pay directly, without involving the insurance companies.

A. A very appropriate thing to do.
B. Appropriate, but not ideal.
C. Inappropriate, but not awful.
D. A very inappropriate thing to do.

In a dissection class, Anna comes to suspect that Martin, another medical student at her table, has removed a piece of anatomy from the cadaver and put it into his pocket.

How **appropriate** are each of the following responses by **Anna** in this situation?

35. Do nothing, because no-one's been harmed.

A. A very appropriate thing to do.

B. Appropriate, but not ideal.

C. Inappropriate, but not awful.

D. A very inappropriate thing to do.

36. Report her suspicions to the anatomy demonstrator.

A. A very appropriate thing to do.

B. Appropriate, but not ideal.

C. Inappropriate, but not awful.

D. A very inappropriate thing to do.

37. Try to confirm with Martin whether he's removed a piece of anatomy from the cadaver and put it into his pocket.

A. A very appropriate thing to do.

B. Appropriate, but not ideal.

C. Inappropriate, but not awful.

D. A very inappropriate thing to do.

38. Ask each of the four other students at the table whether they saw Martin removing a piece of anatomy from the cadaver and putting it into his pocket.

A. A very appropriate thing to do.

B. Appropriate, but not ideal.

C. Inappropriate, but not awful.

D. A very inappropriate thing to do.

39. Ask Martin to turn out his pockets.

A. A very appropriate thing to do.

B. Appropriate, but not ideal.

C. Inappropriate, but not awful.

D. A very inappropriate thing to do.

Dr James is busy taking a history from a stable patient, when the A&E receptionist informs him that a man in the waiting area is getting increasingly angry and agitated. The receptionist appears very anxious.

How **appropriate** are each of the following responses by **Dr James** in this situation?

40. Tell the receptionist not to disturb him while he is engaged with a patient.

A. A very appropriate thing to do.
B. Appropriate, but not ideal.
C. Inappropriate, but not awful.
D. A very inappropriate thing to do.

41. Ask the receptionist to deal with the situation, because it's not strictly a medical matter.

A. A very appropriate thing to do.
B. Appropriate, but not ideal.
C. Inappropriate, but not awful.
D. A very inappropriate thing to do.

42. Ask the receptionist to seek out someone else, because he's currently engaged with a patient.

A. A very appropriate thing to do.
B. Appropriate, but not ideal.
C. Inappropriate, but not awful.
D. A very inappropriate thing to do.

43. Ask the receptionist to call security if she thinks that the man is a threat.

A. A very appropriate thing to do.
B. Appropriate, but not ideal.
C. Inappropriate, but not awful.
D. A very inappropriate thing to do.

44. Go to the reception area, apologise to the angry man, and reassure him that he will be seen as soon as possible.

A. A very appropriate thing to do.
B. Appropriate, but not ideal.
C. Inappropriate, but not awful.
D. A very inappropriate thing to do.

45. Go to the reception area and ask the angry man to leave.

A. A very appropriate thing to do.
B. Appropriate, but not ideal.
C. Inappropriate, but not awful.
D. A very inappropriate thing to do.

Don, Andy and Jo are medical students. Andy feels that Don can be quite bullying towards Jo, frequently criticising her and teasing her for her occasional inability to keep up with the subject matter at medical school.

How **appropriate** are each of the following responses by **Andy** in this situation?

46. Discuss the matter with the academic tutor.

A. A very appropriate thing to do.

B. Appropriate, but not ideal.

C. Inappropriate, but not awful.

D. A very inappropriate thing to do.

47. Discuss the matter with Jo, to determine whether she is bothered by Don's behaviour.

A. A very appropriate thing to do.

B. Appropriate, but not ideal.

C. Inappropriate, but not awful.

D. A very inappropriate thing to do.

48. Discuss the matter with Don, being careful not to suggest that Jo has asked him (Andy) to intervene.

A. A very appropriate thing to do.

B. Appropriate, but not ideal.

C. Inappropriate, but not awful.

D. A very inappropriate thing to do.

49. Start actively criticising Don about any little thing he does wrongly, in order to divert his attention from Jo and teach him what's it's like to be bullied.

A. A very appropriate thing to do.

B. Appropriate, but not ideal.

C. Inappropriate, but not awful.

D. A very inappropriate thing to do.

Sonya is an experienced emergency department physician travelling on a British Airways flight from New York's JFK Airport to London Heathrow. During the journey, a call comes over the public address system, asking whether a doctor is on board to assist with a medical emergency.

How **important** to take into account are the following considerations for **Sonya** when deciding how to respond to the situation?

50. Her level of expertise and competence in emergency healthcare as an emergency department physician.

A. Very important.

B. Important.

C. Of minor importance.

D. Not important at all.

51. Whether she has extra professional indemnity insurance to cover her for non-NHS work.

A. Very important.

B. Important.

C. Of minor importance.

D. Not important at all.

52. How tired she is.

A. Very important.

B. Important.

C. Of minor importance.

D. Not important at all.

Greg is a junior eye surgeon. He has a chesty cough, and after several days of illness he thinks he's developing a chest infection. He considers prescribing himself a short course of oral antibiotics to treat it.

How **important** to take into account are the following considerations for **Greg** when deciding how to respond to the situation?

53. The time this would save Greg.

    A. Very important.

    B. Important.

    C. Of minor importance.

    D. Not important at all.

54. The uncertainty of the diagnosis.

    A. Very important.

    B. Important.

    C. Of minor importance.

    D. Not important at all.

55. Professional guidance around self-prescription.

    A. Very important.

    B. Important.

    C. Of minor importance.

    D. Not important at all.

56. The time this would save Greg's GP, freeing her to see a different patient instead.

    A. Very important.

    B. Important.

    C. Of minor importance.

    D. Not important at all.

57. The risk of increasing antibiotic resistance.

    A. Very important.

    B. Important.

    C. Of minor importance.

    D. Not important at all.

Mike is a fourth-year medical student. While doing a placement in a GP surgery, he becomes concerned about one of the GPs working there. Mike finds him rude and surly to many of his patients, and scathing about them in private after the consultation.

How **appropriate** are each of the following responses by **Mike** in this situation?

58. Discuss his concerns with the GP in question.

A. A very appropriate thing to do.

B. Appropriate, but not ideal.

C. Inappropriate, but not awful.

D. A very inappropriate thing to do.

59. Discuss his concerns with another GP at the practice.

A. A very appropriate thing to do.

B. Appropriate, but not ideal.

C. Inappropriate, but not awful.

D. A very inappropriate thing to do.

60. Discuss his concerns with his fellow medical students.

A. A very appropriate thing to do.

B. Appropriate, but not ideal.

C. Inappropriate, but not awful.

D. A very inappropriate thing to do.

61. Use the practice database to find the patients' contact details and ask them whether they actually felt insulted, before acting further.

A. A very appropriate thing to do.

B. Appropriate, but not ideal.

C. Inappropriate, but not awful.

D. A very inappropriate thing to do.

Johann is a speciality registrar. While on his lunch break in a local public café, he takes a call from work and discusses a patient's case. He takes care not to mention the patient by name, but the conversation is audible to those sitting at neighbouring tables. Jasmine, a consultant surgeon in a different speciality at Johann's hospital, is sitting at one of those tables.

How **appropriate** are each of the following responses by **Jasmine** in this situation?

62. Approach Johann at the café, to point out that while no names were mentioned, someone might still recognise the patient from the case details.

  A. A very appropriate thing to do.
  B. Appropriate, but not ideal.
  C. Inappropriate, but not awful.
  D. A very inappropriate thing to do.

63. Approach Johann later at the hospital, to point out that while no names were mentioned, someone might still recognise the patient from the case details.

  A. A very appropriate thing to do.
  B. Appropriate, but not ideal.
  C. Inappropriate, but not awful.
  D. A very inappropriate thing to do.

64. Talk to Johann's consultant later that day about Johann's behaviour.

  A. A very appropriate thing to do.
  B. Appropriate, but not ideal.
  C. Inappropriate, but not awful.
  D. A very inappropriate thing to do.

65. Ignore the situation, because it's none of her (Jasmine's) business, and, besides, the odds of someone at the café recognising the patient are fairly low.

  A. A very appropriate thing to do.
  B. Appropriate, but not ideal.
  C. Inappropriate, but not awful.
  D. A very inappropriate thing to do.

Tony is a junior doctor, working a busy night shift in a general hospital. He's so busy that he works beyond the end of his shift, seeing a very unwell lady during that time. In his exhaustion, he forgets to order an important diagnostic test. The patient dies overnight, and a serious untoward incident investigation is started.

How **important** to take into account are the following considerations for **investigators** when deciding how to respond to the situation?

66. Tony worked beyond the end of his allotted shift.

    A. Very important.
    B. Important.
    C. Of minor importance.
    D. Not important at all.

67. Whether the missed test contributed to harming the patient.

    A. Very important.
    B. Important.
    C. Of minor importance.
    D. Not important at all.

68. Whether the patient's family complain.

    A. Very important.
    B. Important.
    C. Of minor importance.
    D. Not important at all.

Sandra is a consultant in A&E. She sees a five-year-old boy with a broken arm. It's the third time he's been in A&E with a similar injury over the past two years. Sandra begins to suspect child abuse.

How **important** to take into account are the following considerations for **Sandra** when deciding whether to act on her suspicions?

69. The mother's account of events.

    A. Very important.

    B. Important.

    C. Of minor importance.

    D. Not important at all.

70. The child's account of events.

    A. Very important.

    B. Important.

    C. Of minor importance.

    D. Not important at all.

71. Whether the hospital has a policy on reporting potential child abuse.

    A. Very important.

    B. Important.

    C. Of minor importance.

    D. Not important at all.

Answers

1, D; **2**, D; **3**, D; **4**, A; **5**, A; **6**, B

Discussion:

Signing the register in someone else's name is not only unethical, but could land you and your clinical partner in a lot of trouble. Regardless of the circumstances, signing the register in someone else's name is a very inappropriate thing to do. Therefore, answers 1–3 are all D.

Refusing to sign, underlining that this would be unethical, is appropriate, making answer 4 A. Ideally, though, you also want to make your clinical partner understand why her request is unethical, so answer 5 is also A.

Bringing up the matter with the academic tutor before having had this discussion would be premature and possibly uncalled for, so answer 6 is B.

7, A; **8**, C; **9**, A; **10**, D

Discussion:

The issue of confidentiality is at the heart of this matter, and so it's very important that you should consider it (although this need not mean that you're not going to break confidentiality). Answer 7 is therefore A.

Whether the patient is compliant with her medication is relevant, but not so important in deciding whether to break confidentiality. Answer 8 is therefore C.

The possible consequences of the interaction between alcohol and the patient's medication are very important: if the interaction is potentially fatal, there's a very strong case for breaking confidentiality, so answer 9 is A.

Answer 10 is D, because the patient's opinion of her consultant is unimportant, given that the situation could be a matter of life or death.

11, C; **12**, A; **13**, D; **14**, D

Discussion:

You can't simply let this matter pass, regardless of the circumstances. By passing off his sister's essay as his own, your flatmate is not only damaging his learning, but also gaining an unfair advantage and setting a dangerous precedent — especially for a future medical practitioner. Answers 13 and 14 must therefore be D.

At the same time, to discuss the issue with the ethics lecturer at the soonest opportunity would be premature, and damage your relationship with your flatmate, so answer 11 is C.

What you ought to do, at least in the first instance, is to discuss the issue with your flatmate when he is sober, establish the facts, remind him of the implications and possible consequences of his behaviour, and encourage him to deal with the problem himself. So item 12 is A.

15, D; **16**, B; **17**, A; **18**, A; **19**, D

Discussion:

Regardless of your friendship or of mitigating circumstances, your overriding concern in this case is to protect the safety of the patients that John will be caring for, although you should also have regard for John's welfare, particularly his mental and physical health. This explains answers 17-19.

The tasks that John is due to perform on that day ought not to affect your behaviour, not least because doctors often find themselves involved in unpredictable, emergency situations. So answer 15 is D.

Answer 16 highlights that while John's reputation and career progression are also important, they're not as vital to take into account as the safety of his patients. Having said that, by preventing him from coming into contact with patients and encouraging him to seek help, you are actually protecting his reputation and career.

20, A; **21**, D; **22**, D; **23**, A

Discussion:

To explore Mrs Dickinson's motivations is very appropriate, because it may be that she feels under some obligation to you or that she has ulterior motives in mind. So 20 is A.

To ask Mrs Dickinson to buy you something else instead is inappropriate, particularly if you mean anything more than simple flowers or chocolates (which are deemed to be acceptable gifts). Donating the money to charity is also inappropriate, because money would still change hands. Both make the situation worse, by you accepting the gift, so both 21 and 22 are D.

To politely decline the money by telling Mrs Dickinson that accepting money and valuable gifts is against guidelines is the best ultimate course of action, so item 23 is A. It's also worth noting that some patients, such as those suffering from dementia, might not have the mental capacity to make decisions about their money.

24, A; **25**, A; **26**, A; **27**, D; **28**, A

Discussion:

It's likely that Mrs Jones fears that the administration of the vaccine might lead Noah to develop autism or inflammatory bowel disease. By exploring Mrs Jones's concerns, Dr Aldred could proceed to reassure her that there's no evidence to support a distinct syndrome of MMR-induced autism or inflammatory bowel disease. Answer 24 is therefore A.

Answers 25 and 26 are A because in deciding whether and how strongly to press for the MMR vaccine, Dr Aldred needs primarily to consider the benefits and risks, both for Noah and for the population at large, of receiving the vaccine versus not receiving the vaccine. However, financial incentives for meeting national targets should not be a direct consideration, making item 27 best answered as D.

If Mrs Jones were to insist on refusing the vaccine, then Dr Aldred would have to respect her decision, even if he (and the guidelines) did not agree with it, so 28 is A.

29, A; **30**, D; **31**, B

Discussion:

Having romantic relationships with former patients can seem like a very complex issue, but current professional guidance is actually just a restatement of common sense and good basic ethics.

In brief, guidance says that you shouldn't have romantic relationships with current patients or patients likely to come under your care, and shouldn't use your professional role to create situations where you can take advantage of vulnerable patients. However, if, after some time, you happen to encounter a former patient who is no longer under your care and you then happen to have a relationship with them, that's acceptable.

Item 29 is therefore both appropriate and ideal (answer A), because Ella is attracted to her former patient. Answer 31 is perfectly appropriate but not ideal, for the same reason. Answer 30 is D, because Ella would be inadvertently revealing confidential medical information about the person in front of her group of friends, which includes people who cannot have known that he had been in hospital.

32, A; **33**, D; **34**, A

Discussion:

It's highly unethical to leave the scene of even a minor car accident without leaving some form of contact details so that the damage you caused can be made good. Answer 32 is therefore A, and 33 is D.

At the same time, you are under no ethical or legal obligation to use your insurance policy if a private agreement can be reached instead. Answer 34 is therefore A.

35, D; **36**, B; **37**, A; **38**, C; **39**, D

Discussion:

Although no one has been harmed, to covertly remove a piece of human anatomy from the dissecting room is highly unethical behaviour, so answer 35 is D. If the story came out, it would make people less likely to donate their bodies to medicine. While it's appropriate for Anna to share her suspicions with the anatomy demonstrator, it's best if she tries to verify her suspicions first, and the best way to do this is to speak to Martin (making answer 36 B, and answer 37 A). To ask other students what they saw, while not awful, would risk damaging Martin's reputation among his peers, so answer 38 is C. To ask Martin to turn out his pockets is not Anna's place, making answer 39 D.

40, D; **41**, D; **42**, C; **43**, B; **44**, A; **45**, D

Discussion:

The receptionist is clearly out of her depth and is effectively asking for help. She most likely would not have disturbed Dr James if she felt able to deal with the situation herself, or if someone else had been available to assist her. Because Dr James is occupied with a non-urgent case, he ought to be able to assist his colleague and, hopefully, defuse the situation in the waiting area. These points explain answers 40–42.

Should the situation in the waiting area escalate, it could present a risk both to staff and members of the general public – not to mention to the angry man himself. To go to the reception area and ask the man to leave might inflame the situation, and could also be unfair on the man, who might have legitimate or at least understandable reasons for being angry. Answer 45 is therefore D. To apologise to the angry man and reassure him that he will be seen as soon as possible would be the best course of action (so answer 44 is A) and quite likely to defuse or at least contain the situation. Calling security, while not strictly inappropriate, ought to be a last resort, so answer 43 is B.

46, B; **47**, A; **48**, A; **49**, D

Discussion:

Health professionals should not act in a bullying manner towards each other. They should support each other through difficult times and foster a good team environment. Andy does therefore have a duty to act to resolve this situation. Ideally, he should attempt to verify his impression of the situation by talking to both parties in an unobstrusive way. The answers to both 47 and 48 are therefore A. Going directly to the academic tutor to discuss the situation is appropriate, but because the matter could be successfully resolved without taking that step, it's not ideal, making answer 46 B.

To attempt to turn the tables on Don, to teach him a lesson, is to perpetuate the cycle of abuse and can only make the situation worse, so item 49 is best answered as D.

50, B; **51**, C; **52**, B

Discussion:

The opportunity to undertake good Samaritan acts is thankfully rare. However, doctors have a general duty to help those in need of their services where possible, including in emergency situations when safe to do so. This duty is tempered by doctors' awareness of their own ability to help. Sonya's general qualification as a doctor is therefore vital to take into account, but question 50 asks about her expert knowledge of emergency care, and this is only important rather than vital (B).

Someone's life may be at risk, and this should override any concerns about being insured against negligence tort. It's untrue to say that this shouldn't concern Sonya at all, because doctors have a general duty to be covered against such claims, but being insured is only of minor importance compared with a life potentially hanging in the balance. Answer 51 is therefore C. In fact, British Airways (and most other British transatlantic carriers) will indemnify doctors. And US carriers have to do so by law. You don't need to know this specialist information to answer item 50 correctly, however.

Sonya's tiredness is certainly important, because it may affect her ability to act appropriately under the circumstances. It doesn't override her duty to try to help, so item 52 should be answered as B rather than A, but if another equally qualified and more refreshed doctor is on the flight, that person might be better placed to assist.

53, C; **54**, B; **55**, A; **56**, C; **57**, B

Discussion:

The GMC advises that doctors should not self-prescribe under most practical circumstances. This is obviously vital information, so answer 55 is A. While the UKCAT doesn't expect you to know the GMC's guidance, it's reasonable for you to realise that if there is such guidance, it's of vital importance.

The reasons why the GMC advises that doctors should not normally self-prescribe are that doctors cannot always be confident of their own diagnosis (making item 54 important, and answered as B), and that encouraging it can lead to public distrust in the prescription system, as well as creating a temptation for doctors to self-prescribe addictive substances.

The time it would save Greg and the GP is not completely unimportant; it would potentially help both Greg and the GP work more efficiently. However, this is only of minor importance (answers 53 and 56 being C), because other factors, such as professional guidance, weigh much more strongly.

Finally, antibiotic resistance is a real and growing issue. It's not a vitally important issue in Greg's dilemma, but is part of the reason for getting a GP's opinion on the diagnosis before starting a course of antibiotics. Greg is a trainee eye surgeon, so is not as well placed as a GP to make judgements about starting antibiotics for a presumed chest infection. Therefore, the answer to 57 is B.

58, A; **59**, A; **60**, B; **61**, D

Discussion:

Raising concerns about another doctor who is acting unprofessionally is an important duty. It's certainly very appropriate to discuss the concerns with the GP directly if possible, so answer 58 is A, although for some students the power imbalance between student and GP may make the student feel uncomfortable in doing so. If this is the case, then it's just as appropriate to talk to the GP's colleagues, making answer 59 A as well.

Talking to fellow medical students is not inappropriate, and as long as it's done in a way that respects confidentiality, it may be an appropriate first step to deciding how to act. Answer 60 is therefore B.

Accessing the practice database to find patients' confidential contact details is highly unethical behaviour, regardless of motivation, so answer 61 is D.

62, D; **63**, A; **64**, A; **65**, D

Discussion:

It's certainly very appropriate to talk to Johann about the situation (so 63 is A), but a public café is the wrong setting for such a discussion and may make the situation worse by attracting public attention to it (making 62 D). It's also wrong to simply ignore the problem (so 65 is D), because preserving confidentiality is a key duty of any doctor, and Jasmine has a duty to ensure that Johann learns from this mistake. If Jasmine feels uncomfortable talking directly to Johann about the issue, it would be just as valid to talk to Johann's consultant (making answer 64 A), so that the consultant could discuss it with him in supervision.

66, B; **67**, A; **68**, C

Discussion:

Investigators will have to look into all aspects of the sad death of the patient. Clearly, whether the patient suffered harm as a result of the missed test is of vital importance (so answer 67 is A). It may seem that working beyond the end of your shift to help out when it's busy is a good thing, but most hospitals these days have specific policies against doing this, partly because of employment legislation but also because accidents are more likely to happen when people are working while tired. Tony working beyond the end of his shift is therefore an important consideration, although not vital (answer 66 is B).

69, B; **70**, B; **71**, D

Discussion:

Reporting potential child abuse is vitally important. The accounts of both the mother and child are obviously important, but the fact that Sandra is already worried that this might be child abuse means that their accounts are unlikely to convince her completely. Answers 69 and 70 are therefore only B.

Answer 71 is D because Sandra has a duty to report her concerns irrespective of whether the hospital has a specific policy on doing so. Of course, the steps she takes to raise her concerns may alter, depending on the content of the policy. But she should act on them even if there isn't a specific policy.

Part III
Practice Tests

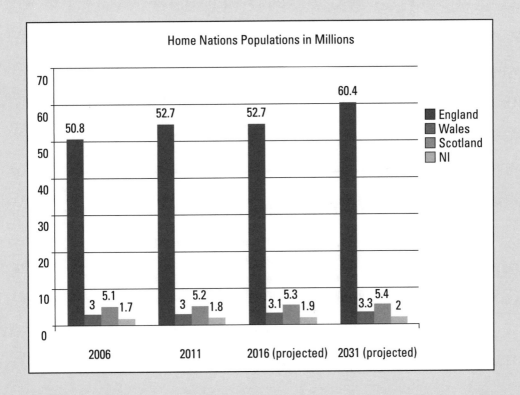

Home Nations Populations in Millions

England
Wales
Scotland
NI

50.8
52.7
52.7
60.4

3 5.1 1.7
3 5.2 1.8
3.1 5.3 1.9
3.3 5.4 2

2006   2011   2016 (projected)   2031 (projected)

For Dummies can help you get started with a huge range of subjects.
Visit www.dummies.com to learn more and do more with *For Dummies*.

In this part . . .

✔ Work your way through two full-sized UKCAT practice tests – against the clock if you can.

✔ Check out the answers and explanations for each test to deepen you understanding of UKCAT.

Chapter 9

Practice Test One

• •

In This Chapter

▶ Working through a complete timed UKCAT practice test

• •

The best way to prepare for the UKCAT test is to do lots of practice questions under timed conditions. In this chapter, we give you a complete practice test, just like the real thing. We recommend that you do the practice test in one session. Make sure that you allow the right amount of time for each part of the test (we show the UKCAT subtest timings in the following table).

Timings for the UKCAT Subtests

Subtest	Time Allowed
Verbal reasoning	22 minutes
Quantitative reasoning	23 minutes
Abstract reasoning	14 minutes
Decision analysis	34 minutes
Situational judgement test	27 minutes

If you have special educational needs and plan to sit the UKCATSEN, give yourself an extra 25 per cent of time. (For the low-down on the UKCATSEN, see Chapter 2.)

In Chapter 10, we give the answers and full explanations for the questions in this practice test.

Verbal Reasoning

Rome in Chaos

(Adapted from *The History of the Decline and Fall of the Roman Empire* by Edward Gibbon)

Pestilence and famine contributed to fill up the measure of the calamities of Rome. The first could be only imputed to the just indignation of the gods; but a monopoly of corn was considered as the immediate cause of the second. The popular discontent at these calamities, after it had long circulated in whispers, broke out in the assembled circus. The people quitted their favourite amusements for the more delicious pleasure of revenge, rushed in crowds towards a palace in the suburbs, one of the emperor's retirements, and demanded, with angry clamours, the head of the public enemy.

Cleander ordered a body of Praetorian cavalry to sally forth and disperse the seditious multitude. The multitude fled with precipitation towards the city, but when the cavalry entered the streets their pursuit was checked by a shower of stones and darts from the roofs and windows of the houses. The foot guards, who had been long jealous of the Praetorians, embraced the party of the people. The tumult became a regular engagement. The Praetorians gave way, oppressed with numbers, and the tide of popular fury returned with redoubled violence against the gates of the palace, where the Emperor Commodus lay, dissolved in luxury and alone, unconscious of the civil war.

Commodus started from his dream of pleasure, and commanded that the head of Cleander should be thrown out to the people. The desired spectacle instantly appeased the tumult, and he might even yet have regained the affection and confidence of his subjects.

1. A corn monopoly was partially responsible for the violence.

   A. True
   B. False
   C. Can't tell

2. Commodus was asleep while the riot was taking place.

   A. True
   B. False
   C. Can't tell

3. The crowd initially routed by cavalry fought back only once then retreated outside the city.

   A. True
   B. False
   C. Can't tell

4. By sacrificing Cleander, Commodus regained the confidence of his subjects.

   A. True
   B. False
   C. Can't tell

Exporting the Format

(Adapted from *The Unauthorized Guide To Doing Business the Jamie Oliver Way* by Trevor Clawson)

Jamie Oliver's television career has taken a new international direction through an agreement to produce a series of six programmes specifically for the US market.

The shows follow Oliver on an odyssey to Huntingdon, West Virginia, a town recognised as one of the most obese and unhealthy in the entire US. During his stay there, Oliver attempts to persuade and encourage the population to adopt a healthier diet.

As in the UK, Oliver has his work cut out. According to the Centers for Disease Control and Prevention, around half the population of the Huntingdon–Ashland metropolitan district are obese, and the area has the highest incidence of heart disease and diabetes in the US. To emphasise the point, in one of Oliver's early encounters – as reported in *The New York Times* – he meets an 8-year-old child suffering from type 2 diabetes and carrying 80 pounds more than her recommended weight.

The US shows follow a long tradition of UK and European reality shows successfully adapted for the US market. If the US show proves a success, it will undoubtedly be re-exported back to the UK, underlining Oliver's global bankability.

5. The first person Oliver met during his TV show was the 8-year-old child with type 2 diabetes mentioned in the passage.

A. True
B. False
C. Can't tell

6. Around half the population of the Huntingdon-Ashland Metropolitan district are obese, with heart disease or diabetes.

A. True
B. False
C. Can't tell

7. British viewers may get to see the programme if it does well in the US.

A. True
B. False
C. Can't tell

8. British reality TV formats can work well in the US.

A. True
B. False
C. Can't tell

Getting to the Bottom Line

(Adapted from *Never Mind the Sizzle . . . Where's the Sausage?* by David J Taylor)

The Simpton's sausages numbers made for sorry reading. The profitability of the core sausage business had been in decline for five years, with the brand trapped in a vicious downward cycle of increasing price promotion, leading to less funds for marketing and innovation, leading to less differentiation, more price promotion, and so on.

In a way, I felt partly responsible for the nightmare we were having, having been part of the sales department's push for more promotional support to protect listings with the key supermarket chains such as Tesco, Sainsbury's and Asda–Walmart.

At the same time, the supermarkets had been busy developing their 'own label' sausage ranges, such as Tesco's Finest and Sainsbury's Taste the Difference.

Our market share had fallen off a cliff, dropping from 35 percent in 1999 to 19 percent in 2006. We had been squashed between the competitively priced supermarket brands at one end, and premium-priced gourmet products at the other, from brands like Duchy Originals and Porkinson.

9. Price is the only determinant of sales in the sausage business.

A. True
B. False
C. Can't tell

10. One way of trying to protect listings with major retailers is with aggressive price promotion.

A. True
B. False
C. Can't tell

11. Squeezed profit margins for Simpton's sausages over the past five years have resulted in less cash available for marketing.

A. True
B. False
C. Can't tell.

12. Over a seven-year period, Simpton's went from a market share of selling more than one in three sausages to fewer than one in five.

A. True
B. False
C. Can't tell

And the Winner is . . .

(Adapted from *The Unauthorized Guide to Doing Business the Simon Cowell Way* by Trevor Clawson)

X Factor is one of the most popular shows on British television and – for good or for ill – it's the only prime-time music show running regularly on any of the major networks. Once upon a time, the BBC's *Top of the Pops* provided the main route to the television audience for mainstream pop acts. With that show long gone, *X Factor* has come to define what British pop music is and how it's presented. And while *Top of the Pops* reflected the whole gamut of popular music, from rap and rock to novelty songs, *X Factor* is about Simon Cowell's vision. He owns the show, owns the successful acts and, if and when he signs them to his label, dictates the course of their careers.

The same is true, to some extent, of Cowell's Syco TV's second big commission for the UK market – *Britain's Got Talent*. As a more generalised talent show, it doesn't necessarily throw up singers or potential recording artists as winners, but has nonetheless proved successful in finding artists for his Syco Music label. These include opera singer Paul Potts, winner of the first show, and Susan Boyle.

The relationship between Syco Music and Syco TV is there on the screen for all to see, but the television production unit is also swelling the coffers of Cowell and joint-venture partner Sony by successfully marketing and selling programmes and their formats around the world.

13. *X Factor* attracts the same audience demographic as *Top of the Pops* used to.

A. True

B. False

C. Can't tell

14. Simon Cowell has a financial interest in both *X Factor* and *Britain's Got Talent.*

A. True

B. False

C. Can't tell

15. Simon Cowell makes more money from *X Factor* than his joint-venture partner Sony does.

A. True

B. False

C. Can't tell

16. Cowell has an interest in Syco TV but not Syco Music.

A. True

B. False

C. Can't tell

Courage

(Adapted from *Plato's Shadow* by Neel Burton)

The man who is willing to hold out in battle in the knowledge that he is in a stronger position is commonly held to be less courageous than the man in the opposite camp who is willing to hold out nonetheless. Yet the second man's behaviour is more foolish than that of the first man, and foolish behaviour is both disgraceful and harmful, whereas courage is always a fine and noble thing. In the Trojan War, Aeneas often took to fleeing on horses, and yet Homer praised him for his knowledge of fear and called him the 'counsellor of fear'. This suggests that courage amounts not to blind recklessness, as most people seem to think, but to the knowledge of the fearful and hopeful in war and, indeed, in every other sphere or situation. Our use of language supports this idea in so far as children and animals, because they have no sense, are never called courageous, but at most fearless.

Fear is produced by anticipated evil things, but not by evil things that have happened or that are happening; in contrast, hope is produced by anticipated good things or by anticipated non-evil things. But for any science of knowledge, there is not one science of the past, one of the present, and one of the future: knowledge of the past, the present and the future are not different types of knowledge, but one and the same. Courage is not merely knowledge of fearful and hopeful things, but knowledge of all things, including those that are in the present and in the past.

17. According to the passage, to what is courage opposed?

A. Fear
B. Foolishness
C. Recklessness
D. Knowledge

18. Which of the following assumptions is central to the author's arguments?

A. Whatever people think must be wrong.
B. Courage is always a fine and noble thing.
C. Children and animals have no sense.
D. Homer can only be right.

19. Which of the following cannot be inferred from the passage?

A. Unless you have knowledge, you can't be said to have courage.
B. You can't fear things that are in the past.
C. The principles of science or knowledge don't change with time.
D. Other virtues such as patience and moderation also amount to knowledge.

20. The author of the passage is least likely to agree with which of the following?

A. People take words and concepts for granted.
B. Careful analysis of the way that words are used can help you to clarify concepts.
C. Popular opinion is usually a good guide to the truth.
D. Courage amounts to the ability to understand the potential risks and benefits of a situation and to act accordingly.

The Raid of John Brown at Harper's Ferry

(Adapted from *The Raid of John Brown at Harper's Ferry as I Saw It* by Samuel Vanderlip Leech)

The town of Harper's Ferry is located in Jefferson County, West Virginia. Lucerne in Switzerland does not excel in romantic grandeur of situation. On its northern front the Potomac sweeps along to pass the national capital, and the tomb of Washington, in its silent flow towards the sea. On its eastern side the Shenandoah hurries to empty its waters into the Potomac, that in perpetual wedlock they may greet the stormy Atlantic. Across the Potomac the Maryland Heights stand out as the tall sentinels of nature. Beyond the Shenandoah are the Blue Ridge Mountains, fringing the westward boundary of Loudon County, Virginia. Between these rivers, and nestling inside of their very confluence, reposes Harper's Ferry. Back of its hills lies the famous Shenandoah Valley, celebrated for its natural scenery, its historic battles and 'Sheridan's Ride'.

At Harper's Ferry, the United States authorities early located an arsenal and an armoury. Captain John Brown believed that if he could secure the arms and ammunition in these buildings, carry them into the fastnesses of the adjacent mountains, and then unfurl the flag of freedom for all slaves who would flock to his standard, the result would be a general uprising of slaves throughout the border states.

21. The author finds Harper's Ferry more beautiful than Lucerne.

   A. True
   B. False
   C. Can't tell

22. Harper's Ferry is bounded by the Shenandoah and the Potomac.

   A. True
   B. False
   C. Can't tell

23. The local slave population was ready to rise up.

   A. True
   B. False
   C. Can't tell

24. Captain Brown intended to make his stand in the town, after securing the arsenal and armoury.

   A. True
   B. False
   C. Can't tell

Something Wonderful

(Adapted from *The Railway Children* by Edith Nesbit)

'I wish something would happen,' said the eldest child, Bobbie, dreamily, 'something wonderful.' Now, curiously enough, this was just what happened.

The old gentleman, who was very well known and respected at his particular station, had got there early that morning, and he had waited at the door where the young man stands holding the interesting machine that clips the tickets, and he had said something to every single passenger who passed through that door. And after nodding to what the old gentleman had said – and the nods expressed every shade of surprise, interest, doubt, cheerful pleasure and grumpy agreement – each passenger had gone onto the platform and read one certain part of his newspaper. And when the passengers got into the train, they had told the other passengers who were already there what the old gentleman had said, and then the other passengers had also looked at their newspapers and seemed very astonished and, mostly, pleased. Then, when the train passed the fence where the three children were, newspapers and hands and handkerchiefs were waved madly, till all that side of the train was fluttery with white like the pictures of the King's Coronation in the biograph at Maskelyne and Cook's. To the children it almost seemed as though the train itself was alive, and was at last responding to the love that they had given it so freely and so long.

25. Bobbie knew something wonderful was going to happen.

A. True

B. False

C. Can't tell

26. The old gentlemen ensured that many train passengers waved at the children from their windows.

A. True

B. False

C. Can't tell

27. The children loved seeing the train, even before the passengers waved back at them.

A. True

B. False

C. Can't tell

28. The children knew why everyone was waving at them.

A. True

B. False

C. Can't tell

Social Commerce

(Adapted from *Socialnomics* by Erik Qualman)

Social commerce is upon us. What is social commerce exactly? It's a term that encompasses the transactional, search and marketing components of social media. Social commerce harnesses the simple idea that people value the opinion of other people. What this truly means is that in the future we will no longer seek products and services; rather, they will find us. Nielsen reports that 78 per cent of people trust their peers' opinions. This is neither a new concept, nor new to the Web.

What's new is that social media makes it so much easier to disseminate information. As the success of social media proves, people enjoy spreading information. This explains the popularity of Twitter, Foursquare, Gowalla, and so forth. These tools and products enable users to inform their friends what they are doing every minute of the day (I'm having an ice cream cone; check out this great article; listening to keynote speaker; etc.). Twitter is interesting from the standpoint that its popularity began with older generations, and time will tell how much of Generation Y and Z embrace Twitter. This is the exact opposite trend of Facebook, which was originally popular with the younger generations and then Generation X and Baby Boomers started to get engaged.

The most popular feature of Facebook and LinkedIn is status updates. Status updates enable users to continuously brag, boast, inform and vent to everyone in their network.

29. Social commerce is a buzzword for how social media interacts with business.

    A. True
    B. False
    C. Can't tell

30. Facebook was originally popular because younger people are less socially inhibited than older generations.

    A. True
    B. False
    C. Can't tell

31. Most sharing on social media is, in fact, a form of bragging.

    A. True
    B. False
    C. Can't tell

32. Research suggests that most people trust their peers' opinions.

    A. True
    B. False
    C. Can't tell

Chinese Water Crisis

(Adapted from *An Introduction to the Chinese Economy* by Rongxing Guo)

China now faces almost all of the problems related to water resources that are faced by countries across the globe. China's rapid economic growth, industrialisation and urbanisation have outpaced infrastructural investment and management capacity, and have created widespread problems of water scarcity. In the areas of the North China Plain, where about half of China's wheat and corn is grown and there are extensive peach orchards, drought is an ever-looming threat. With one-fifth of the world's population, China has only 8 per cent of the fresh water. China's annual renewable water reserves were about 2.8 trillion cubic meters, which ranked it fifth in the world, behind Brazil, Russia, Canada and Indonesia, but ahead of the US. However, in terms of per capita availability of water reserves, China has one of the lowest in the world – barely one-quarter of the world average.

In the coming decades, China will be under severe water stress, as defined by the international standard, and there is already growing competition for water between communities, sectors of the economy and individual provinces.

33. China will be unable to adequately manage its limited water supply.

  A. True

  B. False

  C. Can't tell

34. China has 8 per cent of the water it needs, by international standards.

  A. True

  B. False

  C. Can't tell

35. China has less water than it needs, by international standards.

  A. True

  B. False

  C. Can't tell

36. The North China Plain is a major agricultural centre in China.

  A. True

  B. False

  C. Can't tell

The Dead Rise

(Adapted from *The Proper Care and Feeding of Zombies* by Mac Montandon)

In 2009, a small group of highly motivated Canadian mathematicians and researchers took up the humanitarian cause of modelling an infectious zombie outbreak.

The basic equation for determining the rate of a zombie outbreak contained three variables: Susceptibles, Zombies and Removed. The first two categories should be clear enough, and Removed simply refers to dead humans. The creators introduced a special parameter to account for Removed humans who subsequently become Zombies, and another one to allow for Zombies to be Removed by means of 'removing the head or destroying the brain'.

The results are chilling. If no action is taken, the zombie outbreak will overtake a city of half a million people in roughly four days. However, if counter-strikes by humans are permitted, it's possible for humans to win and eradicate the zombies within just ten days. This assumes that the attacks are 'sufficiently frequent, with increasing force, and that the available resources can be mustered in time'.

37. Canadian researchers are interested in zombie outbreaks.

   A. True
   B. False
   C. Can't tell

38. Zombies cannot be killed, because they are already undead.

   A. True
   B. False
   C. Can't tell

39. Zombie outbreaks take just days to overwhelm population centres.

   A. True
   B. False
   C. Can't tell

40. Zombies cannot be defeated through superior firepower.

   A. True
   B. False
   C. Can't tell

Understanding Oracles

(Adapted from 'Plato: Letters to My Son' by Neel Burton)

Overcome by their feuding, the citizens of Delos had turned to the Delphic oracle for divine assistance, and the priestess had advised them to double the size of their altar to Apollo. In accordance with their interpretation of the oracular pronouncement, they set out to build another altar with sides twice the length of the original one, but, if anything, their problems only got worse. When they wrote for Plato's opinion, the philosopher replied that the oracle may have meant doubling the volume rather than doubling the lengths of the sides, in which case their new altar, which stood at eight times the volume of the original one, was four times too big. Plato added that, since no one knew the method for calculating the length of side required for doubling the volume of a cube, the gods might in fact have been telling them to take up the study of mathematics and philosophy so as to moderate their passions. Failing that, they could always try building a third altar identical to the first and setting it beside the first or on top of it; but in either case, the altar would no longer be a cube and the gods would probably disregard their efforts and maybe even take affront at their dupery.

41. Which of the following is the best statement of the potential problem with the Delians' new altar?

A. Its sides are too long.

B. It's four times the volume of the original one.

C. It's eight times too big.

D. It isn't double the size of the old altar.

42. According to the text, in his reply to the Delians, Plato made all of the following suggestions except:

A. Build an altar that is only approximately twice the volume of the first.

B. Try building another altar identical to the first and setting it on top of the first.

C. Try building another altar identical to the first and setting it beside the first.

D. Take up the study of mathematics and philosophy.

43. Which of the following can be inferred from the passage:

A. Plato's reply to the Delians is tongue in cheek.

B. The Delians thought that Plato might take their problem seriously.

C. Had the Delians known the method for doubling the volume of a cube, their feuding would have come to an end.

D. The method for doubling the volume of a cube has since been discovered.

44. Which statement is least likely to be true?

A. The Delians had faith in the Delphic oracle.

B. The Delians valued Plato's opinion.

C. Plato understood the principles of geometry.

D. Even before writing to Plato, the Delians understood in what way they had misinterpreted the oracular pronouncement.

Quantitative Reasoning

FTSE All-share Index Market Capitalisations

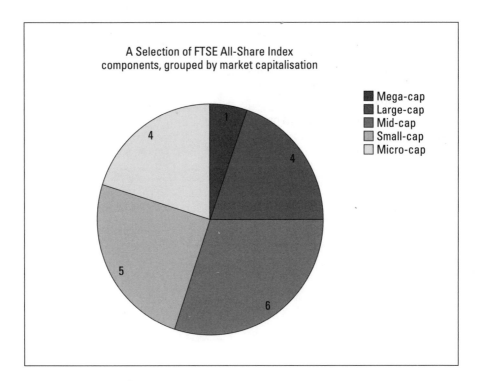

A Selection of FTSE All-Share Index
components, grouped by market capitalisation

- Mega-cap
- Large-cap
- Mid-cap
- Small-cap
- Micro-cap

Market capitalisation is a measure of how large a company is. It's calculated by multiplying the share price by the number of shares in circulation. Companies can be grouped into categories based on the size of their market capitalisation, or 'cap' for short. The largest companies are the mega-caps, followed by large caps, mid-caps, small caps and micro-caps. A selection of companies listed on the Stock Exchange were analysed, and the chart in the figure was created.

1. What percentage of companies are at least large caps in size?

   (A) 5% (B) 20% (C) 25%
   (D) 30% (E) 45%

2. What's the ratio of large caps to micro-caps?

   (A) 1:5 (B) 1:1 (C) 2:1
   (D) 1:4 (E) 1:5

3. Two large caps merge, creating a new single mega-cap company. What's the approximate new percentage of mega caps?

   (A) 5.0% (B) 5.3% (C) 10.0%
   (D) 10.5% (E) 15.0%

4. The mega-cap featured in the initial study is Royal Dutch Shell, a global company with an approximate market capitalisation of £165 billion in 2010. Assuming its share price has fallen by 15% since then, what's its current approximate market capitalisation in billions of US dollars? (Assume £1 = $1.63.)

   (A) 132 (B) 140 (C) 165
   (D) 215 (E) 229

Conflict in Afghanistan

British Fatalities in Afghanistan in 2010	
Month	*Number of Fatalities*
January	6
February	15
March	12
April	3
May	8
June	20
July	16
August	7
September	6
October	4
November	3
December	3

5. Approximately what percentage of fatalities took place up to the end of June?

(A) 50%   (B) 62%   (C) 64%
(D) 78%   (E) 80%

6. If you were a soldier in Afghanistan, approximately how many times greater were your chances of dying in the first half of the year compared with the second half, working solely from the statistics in Table 9-2?

(A) 1.64   (B) 1.78   (C) 2.00
(D) 3.49   (E) 3.50

7. What was the mean number of British deaths per month in Afghanistan in 2010? Round your answer to one decimal place.

(A) 3.0   (B) 5.3   (C) 8.3
(D) 8.6   (E) 12.0

8. In the deadliest month, by what percentage did deaths exceed the modal average, to the nearest whole per cent?

(A) 15%   (B) 380%   (C) 433%
(D) 567%   (E) 667%

Top Flight Material

The table shows the 20 teams playing in the Premier League in the 2011–2012 season, together with the total number of years for which they've played in the top division of English football.

Premiership Clubs' Top-tier Years							
Arsenal	95	Everton	109	Newcastle United	81	Swansea City	3
Aston Villa	101	Fulham	23	Norwich City	22	Tottenham Hotspur	71
Blackburn Rovers	72	Liverpool	97	Queen's Park Rangers	22	West Bromwich Albion	73
Bolton Wanderers	73	Manchester City	83	Stoke City	56	Wigan Athletic	7
Chelsea	77	Man United	87	Sunderland	81	Wolves	63

John, a keen football statistician, decides to group the teams into categories based on how many seasons they've been in the top flight, and draws up the table shown in this table.

John's Table of Premiership Clubs	
Football Royalty (90+ seasons)	4
Aristocrats (70–89 seasons)	9
Bourgeoisie (20–69 seasons)	5
New Boys (19 or fewer seasons)	2

9. Is there anything wrong with John's table?

A. One too many in Football Royalty
B. One too many in the Aristocrats
C. One too few in the Bourgeoisie
D. One too few in the New Boys
E. No – his table is correct

10. If all the current members of the top three categories remain in the Premiership for another ten years, how many members of the Aristocrats will there be then?

(A) 5　(B) 6　(C) 8
(D) 10　(E) 12

11. Returning to the present day, what's the arithmetic mean number of seasons of top flight status held by the Football Royalty clubs? You may round your answer to the nearest whole number of seasons.

    (A) 98 (B) 100 (C) 101
    (D) 105 (E) 122

12. How many more years will it take Wigan Athletic to become Bourgeoisie, assuming that the club is relegated out of the Premier League twice during that time and it takes it a season in the Championship each time to return to the Premier League?

    (A) 9 (B) 13 (C) 14
    (D) 15 (E) 17

Ryding High

Selection to the USA Ryder Cup Golf team is done through a points system. Players collect points based on how they do in tournaments throughout the year. The points of the top-20 players can be found in the table.

Ryder Cup Points				
331	194	408	360	293
803	220	314	163	364
164	390	766	364	184
330	129	330	291	141

13. The top eight players qualify automatically for inclusion in the team. What's the minimum current score that qualifies?

(A) 331 (B) 330 (C) 314
(D) 293 (E) 291

14. What's the range of points?

(A) 625 (B) 637 (C) 662
(D) 673 (E) 674

15. What percentage of the top 20 players will qualify with a cut-off score of 295?

(A) 45% (B) 50% (C) 55%
(D) 60% (E) 65%

16. To the nearest whole per cent, by what percentage does the average point score of the bottom five players have to increase to meet a 295-point cut-off?

(A) 12% (B) 39% (C) 56%
(D) 89% (E) 100%

Speed Test

Items 17–20 refer to the Nürburgring Nordschleife car test track located in Germany.

Nürburgring test times are based on a 20.6-km lap, and times are given in a minutes and seconds format such that 8:55 is 8 minutes and 55 seconds, for example. Speeds are commonly reported in kilometres per hour (km/h) or miles per hour (mph).

If needed, you may assume that 1 mile = 1.6 km.

17. The fastest car around the Nürburgring was the Radical SR8 LM, recording a lap time of 6:48. What was its average speed in miles per hour, to the nearest whole number?

(A) 12   (B) 114   (C) 162
(D) 181   (E) 182

18. The Pagani Zonda F Clubsport took 33:04 to complete three laps. Assuming that 652 seconds was lost due to mechanical problems and time spent recovering from these problems, what would have been its average lap time without these issues?

(A) 0:74   (B) 7:24   (C) 7:40
(D) 11:01   (E) 22:12

19. The Radical mentioned in question 17 weighs just 680 kg. The Zonda mentioned in question 18 weighs 1,210 kg. If Zonda's maximum power is 650 horsepower (hp), what approximately does the Radical need to put out to maintain the same maximal power-to-weight ratio as the Zonda?

(A) 365 hp   (B) 366 hp   (C) 368 hp
(D) 382 hp   (E) 1157 hp

20. The Zonda now does three fresh laps. The first lap manages an average speed of 120 mph, the second a lap time of 7:23, and the third is 5% quicker than the first. What's the approximate average speed of the Zonda across these three laps of the Nürburgring?

(A) 3 km/s   (B) 117 km/h   (C) 117 mph
(D) 185 mph (E) 187 mph

Population Demographics

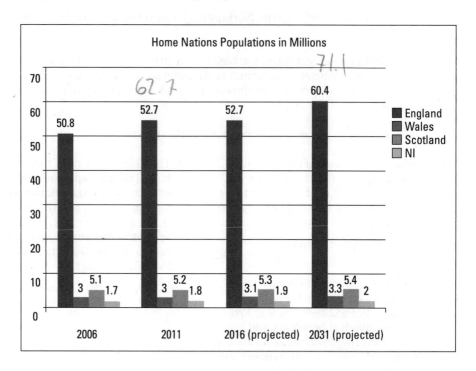

The figure shows the changing population of the UK home nations, in millions, including projections for 2016 and 2031.

21. In 2011, what's the ratio of the English to the populations of the rest of the home nations?

    (A) 1:1.19   (B) 1:1.20   (C) 1.24:1
    (D) 5.18:1   (E) 5.27:1

22. Which of the following statements is supported by the information in the chart?

    A. The Northern Irish population is gradually falling, over the period charted.

    B. On average, the Scottish population is increasing faster than the English population between 2006 and 2031.

    C. The English make up a greater proportion of the total population in 2031 than in 2011.

    D. The Welsh population is projected to increase by approximately 10% between 2016 and 2031.

    E. By 2016, the English and Scottish populations will represent less than 90% of the overall population of the home nations.

23. What's the approximate overall percentage increase in the population of the home nations in 2031 compared with 2011?

    (A) 10.2%   (B) 13.4%   (C) 14.6%
    (D) 17.3%   (E) 18.9%

24. What's the range in millions between the English population and the Welsh population across the entire period charted?

    (A) 9.6   (B) 55.3   (C) 57.1
    (D) 57.4   (E) 58.7

Well-Heeled

James is just starting his career, and decides to buy three pairs of shoes to suit any basic professional need (black plain cap-toe oxfords, dark brown wingtip oxfords and burgundy penny loafers).

He is undecided about whether to buy high-quality but expensive Northampton Classics or cheaper but limited-lifespan Mass Market shoes, so draws up these two tables to compare the costs and help him decide.

Northampton Classics	
Pair of shoes	*£650*
Factory recrafting and resoling (required every five years; can be done a maximum of three times per shoe)	£120 per pair
High-quality polish (total annual cost)	£20
Lasted shoe trees (pair)	£50
Expected lifetime, with good upkeep	20 years per pair

Mass Market Shoes	
Pair of shoes	*£75*
Cheap polish (total annual cost)	£5
Cheap shoe trees (pair)	£10
Expected lifetime, with good upkeep	2 years per pair

25. How much will it cost James to wear Northampton Classics over a 40-year career, assuming that he can reuse the old shoe trees in any new pairs of shoes he needs to buy over that career?

(A) £5,060 (B) £6,210 (C) £7,010
(D) £7,160 (E) £7,730

26. How much will it cost him to wear Mass Market shoes over the same career? (Assume that the cheaper shoe trees will break and need to be replaced once every 20 years.)

(A) £1,760 (B) £4,560 (C) £4,565
(D) £4,730 (E) £4,760

27. Which of the following statements is false?

A. Northampton Classics are more expensive over a career lifetime than mass market shoes.

B. If cost is the only determinant of purchase, James should buy Mass Markets.

C. If James finds the aesthetic value and craftsmanship of Northampton Classics to be superior to that of Mass Market shoes, he may find them worth spending extra money on.

D. The annual cost of wearing Northampton Classics is £175.25.

E. The annual cost of wearing Mass Market shoes is £110.

28. James decides to buy Northampton Classics, but decides to start with four pairs of shoes instead of three, and for that fourth pair adds dark brown Chelsea boots to his collection. This addition reduces the frequency of wearing of each pair and so proportionally reduces the required frequency of resoling. If resoling is the limiting factor determining the overall lifespan of the shoe, for how many years will each pair now last?

(A) 22.5 (B) 24.3 (C) 25.5
(D) 26.7 (E) 30.3

Hitting the Sales

The British Chambers of Commerce hires a market research firm to study how the shopping habits of the public vary in response to a Bank of England interest rate cut of 50 basis points. The researchers compare shoppers with variable mortgages with those without mortgages (or with fixed-rate mortgages) and measure how many of each group increase their weekly discretionary expenditure by at least 10% in the aftermath of the rate cut. This table shows the effect of monetary policy on shopping habits

Effect of Monetary Policy on Shopping Habits			
	Variable Mortgage Holders	Fixed/No Mortgage Holders	Total
Would not increase expenditure by 10%+	52	89	141
Would increase expenditure by 10%+	133	111	244

29. Approximately, what are the odds of a variable-mortgage holder increasing expenditure by at least 10% compared with people who do not hold a variable mortgage?

(A) 1:1   (B) 3:2   (C) 2:1
(D) 3:1   (E) 5:1

30. What percentage of variable-mortgage holders increase their expenditure by at least 10%? Round your answer to the nearest whole per cent.

(A) 21%   (B) 39%   (C) 55%
(D) 72%   (E) 256%

31. What's the difference between the proportion of people who increase expenditure by at least 10% and who are variable-mortgage holders compared with the proportion who increase expenditure by at least 10% but are fixed/no-mortgage holders?

(A) 0.16   (B) 0.18   (C) 0.56
(D) 0.72   (E) 1.20

32. What's the chance that a person selected at random from the study sample has neither a variable mortgage nor increases their expenditure by at least 10% in response to the Bank of England base rate cut?

(A) 13.5%   (B) 23.1%   (C) 28.8%
(D) 34.5%   (E) 37.4%

In at the Deep End

Preparation for the London 2012 Olympics included the design of a new swimming pool to meet FINA long-course standards. The dimensions of such a swimming pool are shown schematically in the following figure.

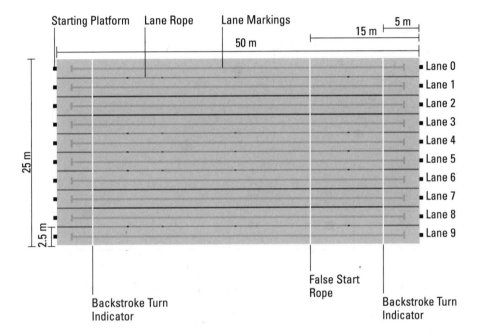

33. Assuming an average depth of 2 metres, what's the total internal surface area of the empty pool in m²?

(A) 1,250 m²   (B) 1,550 m²   (C) 2,500 m²
(D) 2,800 m²   (E) 5,300 m²

34. The pool needs to be tiled. As well as the internal surface area, the pool also needs to be tiled to a border that extends a further 0.5 metres in both length and width beyond the pool's edge. If each tile is 10 cm × 10 cm, how many tiles are required in total?

(A) 7,600   (B) 147,400
(C) 155,000   (D) 162,600   (E) 162,700

35. Pale blue tiles cost 15p each and will be used for most of the pool, but 2,500 tiles need to be dark blue, and these cost 18p per tile. Another 7,500 tiles need to be non-slip and cost 30p each. What's the total cost of the tiles?

(A) £24,390   (B) £24,690
(C) £25,590   (D) £27,090   (E) £48,780

36. It takes a tiler five minutes to lay a tile. Assuming that ten people work a simultaneous eight-hour tiling day and don't interfere in each other's work, on what day do they complete the entire job?

A. The 169th day
B. The 170th day
C. The 504th day
D. The 1,694th day
E. The 2,033rd day

Abstract Reasoning

To which set, if either, does each of the test shapes (Q1 to Q5) belong?

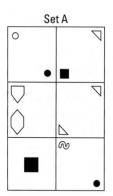

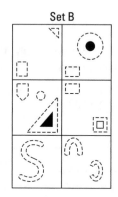

Q1  Q2   Q3  Q4  Q5

To which set, if either, does each of the test shapes (Q6 to Q10) belong?

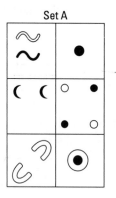

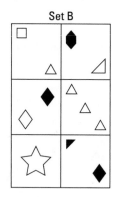

Q6  Q7  Q8  Q9  Q10

To which set, if either, does each of the test shapes (Q11 to Q15) belong?

Set A   Set B

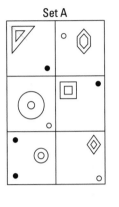   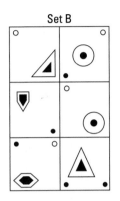

Q11   Q12   Q13   Q14   Q15

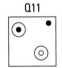 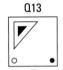 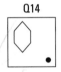 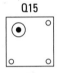

16. Which of the following belongs to Set A?

Set A   Set B

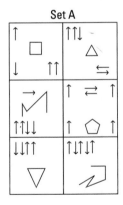   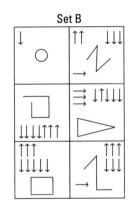   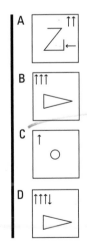

17. Which of the following belongs to Set B?

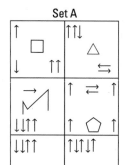

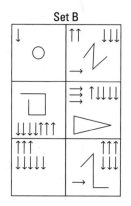

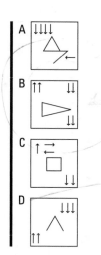

18. Which figure completes the statement?

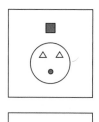

is to

as

is to

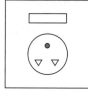

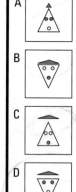

19. Which figure completes the series?

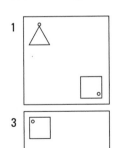

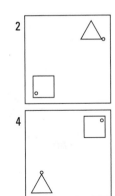

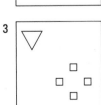

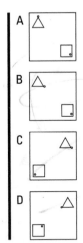

20. Which figure completes the series?

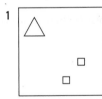

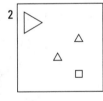

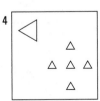

To which set, if either, does each of the test shapes (Q21 to Q25) belong?

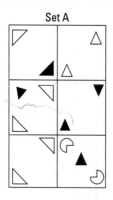

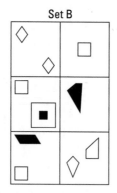

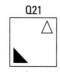

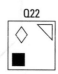

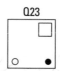

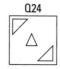

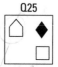

Q21 Q22 Q23 Q24 Q25

To which set, if either, does each of the test shapes (Q26 to Q30) belong?

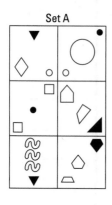

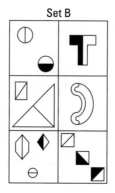

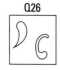

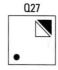

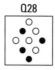

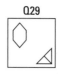

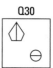

Q26 Q27 Q28 Q29 Q30

To which set, if either, does each of the test shapes (Q31 to Q35) belong?

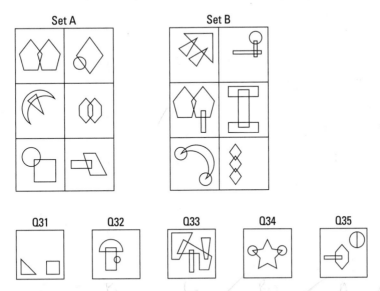

To which set, if either, does each of the test shapes (Q36 to Q40) belong?

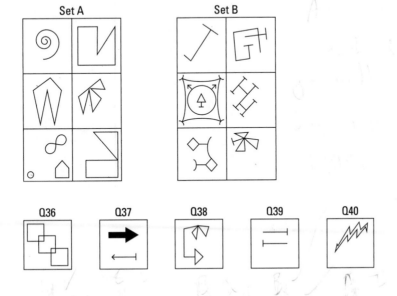

41. Which figure completes the series?

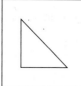

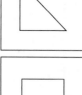

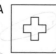

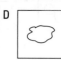

42. Which figure completes the series?

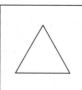

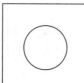

43. Which figure completes the series?

1

2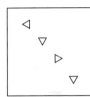

A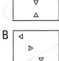

3

4

B

C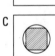

D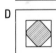

44. Which figure completes the series?

1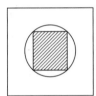

2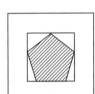

3

4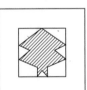

45. Which figure completes the statement?

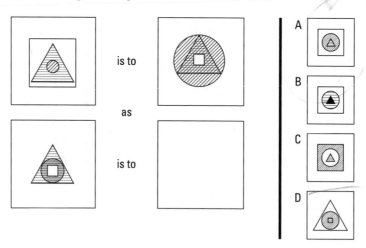

To which set, if either, does each of the test shapes (Q46 to Q50) belong?

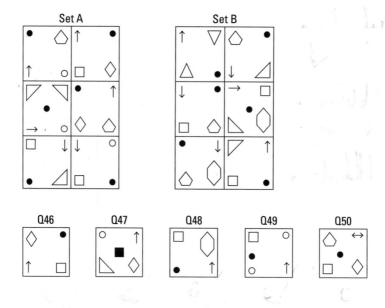

51. Which of the following belongs to Set A?

Set A   Set B   A   △
                                  ○
                                  ○
                                  ◇
                                  □

                              B   □
                                  ○
                                  ○
                                  △
                                  ◇

                              C   □
                                  ◇
                                  ○
                                  ○
                                  △

                              D   ○
                                  △
                                  □
                                  ○
                                  ◇

52. Which of the following belongs to Set B?

Set A   Set B   A   □
                                  ◇
                                  ○
                                  △
                                  ○

                              B   ○
                                  □
                                  △
                                  ○
                                  ◇

                              C   ○
                                  △
                                  ○
                                  ◇
                                  □

                              D   ◇
                                  ○
                                  □
                                  ○
                                  △

This is wrong!

53. Which of the following belongs to Set A?

Set A   Set B

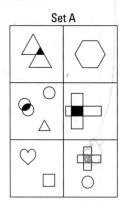
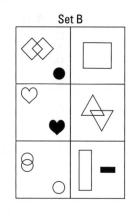
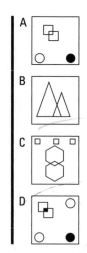

54. Which of the following belongs to Set B?

Set A   Set B

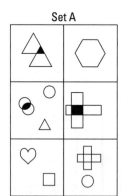
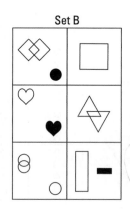
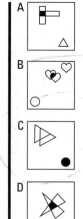

55. Which figure completes the series?

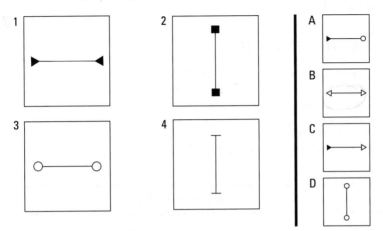

Decision Analysis

The Turin Codex

Legend tells of a mysterious and powerful organisation called the Penumbra
Syndicate, responsible for influencing world history down through the ages.
Little progress was made in understanding the strange system of codes
through which Syndicate members are said to communicate until the recent
dazzling archaeological discovery of the Turin codex, which reveals the
symbolic basis for at least part of the code.

The Turin Codex

Nouns	Verbs	Adjectives	Operator
I = O	Kill = 🔥	Rich = ✡	Positive = 👍
You = ●	Talk = 📖	Poor = ❄	Negative = 👎
He = ■	Pay = ✉	Angry = ☹	Quickly = ☞
King = 🐏	Run = ♉	Calm = ☺	Slowly = 🐌
Pope = ✝	Sail = ♒	Brave = 🌶	Now = ♌
Queen = ♍	Ride = ♐	Cowardly = 🖐	Then = ⌛
Cardinal = ♎	Take = ➑		Conditional = ♎
Knight = ⚑	Burn = ♋		
Peasant = 💧			
Home = ❖			

Armed with the codex, your task is to decipher the following messages
written in the Penumbra Syndicate's code, convert some others into
Penumbra code, and so save the world from the syndicate's malign and
pervasive influence!

1. What's the best interpretation of the following Penumbra message?

   △, ⚺ 💣 , ᎶᎧ

   A. The cardinal will kill the king.
   B. The cardinal has killed the king.
   C. The king will kill the cardinal.
   D. The king has talked to the cardinal.
   E. The king might kill the cardinal.

2. What's the best interpretation of the following Penumbra message?

   ♍, ⚺ 📖, ᎶᎧ, ✉, (O ●)

   A. The king will pay the queen.
   B. The king will persuade the queen to talk to us.
   C. The queen will persuade the king to pay us.
   D. The queen will talk to the king.
   E. The queen will tell the king to fight.

3. What's the best interpretation of the following Penumbra message?

   ✝, ⤢, △ △

   A. The Pope fights his cardinals.
   B. The Pope rides to meet his cardinals.
   C. The Pope bribes his cardinals.
   D. The cardinals plot against the Pope.
   E. The cardinals plot against each other to become Pope.

4. What's the best interpretation of the following Penumbra message?

   ♝ ♝, ♌ ♟

   A. The knights will win the battle.
   B. No knights fought in the previous war.
   C. Knights and bishops will fight together.
   D. The knights won't fight us today.
   E. No knight will dare to challenge the king.

5. What's the best interpretation of the following Penumbra message?

   ♍, ☹, ᎶᎧ, ☞ ♟, ☹ (💣 💣)

   A. The queen is furious at the king's rapid retreat from battle.
   B. The king was routed in the battle.
   C. The queen and king were forced to flee the battle.
   D. No king would leave his queen to be lost in battle.
   E. Defeating the queen is the fastest way to beat the king.

6. What's the best way to translate the following into Penumbra code?

   Bribe the Pope to defy the king.

   A. ✉, ✝, ☹ 📖, ᎶᎧ
   B. ✝, ☹ 📖, ✉ ᎶᎧ
   C. ♝, ✝, ☹ 📖, ᎶᎧ
   D. 💣, ☹ 📖, ✉, ᎶᎧ
   E. ☹ 📖, 💣, ✝, ᎶᎧ

7. What's the best interpretation of the following Penumbra message?

♦♦,♎(❽℗) ● ✉

A. The bribed peasants will lie to you.
B. The peasants will kill the knight if you bribe them.
C. The peasants will revolt if you bribe them.
D. The peasants may not choose to take your bribe.
E. The bribed peasants will commit regicide.

8. What's the best interpretation of the following Penumbra message?

✿(℞℞),☷☺,↝

A. The knights need a rich king.
B. The king will pay his knights handsomely.
C. The knights get rich by killing the king.
D. Wealthy knights will remain loyal to the Pope.
E. Rich knights will remain loyal to the king.

9. What's the best interpretation of the following Penumbra message?

✝,☺📖,☄℗♙,⌖

A. The Pope calmly ordered the execution of the rebel cardinal by burning at the stake.
B. The cardinal ordered his pope to be executed.
C. The Pope furiously ordered that his rebellious cardinal be burned to death.
D. The Pope demanded the death of all renegade cardinals.
E. The Pope fumed as he excommunicated the rebel cardinal.

10. What's the best interpretation of the following Penumbra message?

♦♦,♠⊗,☺(❖❖),℗(℞℞)

A. The peasants bravely fought the knights away from their village.
B. The brave peasants took the evil knight's castle.
C. The peasants fought bravely to defend their homes from the evil knights.
D. The peasants were terrified but still fought off the evil knights.
E. The evil knights charged the brave peasants.

11. What's the best interpretation of the following Penumbra message?

○✉,● ♒,Ravenna,☷☄♙

A. Sailing to Ravenna with the cardinal can be lethal.
B. The Cardinal of Ravenna kills all who arrive at his port.
C. The Cardinal of Ravenna hires sailors as assassins.
D. I'll pay you to sail to Ravenna and kill the cardinal there.
E. Paying the Cardinal of Ravenna is the only way to avoid death.

12. Penumbra messages are often signed with the following inscription.

(○ ●)☺(↝✝)

What's the best interpretation of this phrase?

A. From the shadows, we rule.
B. We control kings, popes and peasants.
C. We subdue both king and Pope.
D. Neither king nor Pope can defeat us.
E. The king will bow before us.

13. What's the best interpretation of the following Penumbra message?

   ⚑◆, ⚘(☹ ⚰※)

   A. The peasant fought the knight.
   B. The knight and his squire fight bravely.
   C. The knight and his entourage fought off the Pope.
   D. The knight carried his squire into battle.
   E. The knight fought his serfs.

14. What's the best interpretation of the following Penumbra message?

   ᧞, 📖, ☺, ☺(᧞ ❖)

   A. The king burned his city to the ground.
   B. The king was burned to death in his city.
   C. The city burned around the invading king.
   D. The invaders ordered the king's city to be torched.
   E. The king ordered a scorched-earth policy to protect his city.

15. What's the best interpretation of the following Penumbra message?

   ●⚔☞, ᧞

   A. Ride to the king as fast as you can!
   B. The king flees from you.
   C. Let the king ride to meet you.
   D. The king's cavalry is swifter than you are.
   E. You can outrun the king's mounted troops.

16. For this question, you may assume that the Pope lives in the Vatican City. Use the Turin codes to encode the following into a message that the Penumbra Syndicate will think is from *its* own operative.

   Burn the Vatican City immediately!

   A. ♰, ☺♌
   B. ♰❖, ☺☞
   C. ♰❖, ☺⚰
   D. ✪♰❖, ☺♌
   E. ♰❖, ☺♌

17. What's the best interpretation of the following Penumbra message?

   (○●)(⛎♔), ♌(○, ●, ■)

   A. I'm trapped – you must get help now.
   B. We're trapped – call for back-up immediately.
   C. We're trapped; it's now every man for himself.
   D. Don't move – I'll come to help you.
   E. We must all remain perfectly still.

18. What's the best interpretation of the following Penumbra message?

   ⚑(●●), ○⚰(☹ ⚰※)

   A. You coward – I won't become angry with you.
   B. I won't become a coward like you.
   C. I'll kill all cowards.
   D. You're all cowards; I'll fight again another day.
   E. Cowardly behaviour does not save you from me.

19. What's the best interpretation of the following Penumbra message?

♎ (᨞☷❋), (O●)❽ᵭ

A. The cowardly king won't stop me.
B. If we bankrupt the king, we may still win.
C. The king is poor but I'm not.
D. The king will pay me enough to no longer be poor.
E. The king is generous while I'm a thief.

20. What's the best interpretation of the following Penumbra message?

◆◆, ✉ᵭᵭ,᨞✝

A. The peasants stole from the king and the Pope.
B. The king stole from the peasants to give to the church.
C. The church taxed the peasants to pay the king.
D. The Pope stole the people's money to bribe the king.
E. The peasants are taxed excessively by both church and state.

21. What's the best interpretation of the following Penumbra message?

♍⊞✉, 📖,⚱,♇📖,♍(᨞(♇ᵭ))

A. The queen paid the cardinal to keep her affair with the king's chief knight a secret.
B. The cardinal's refusal to talk to the queen led to an uprising by the knights.
C. The queen paid the cardinal to promote the king's knight-in-chief.
D. The queen paid the cardinal to arrange for the king to kill his chief nobleman.
E. The king and queen arranged for the knights to bribe the cardinal.

22. The Turin codex is an incomplete portion of modern Penumbra Syndicate code. In particular, the code has been added to over the centuries to include symbols for things that simply didn't exist when the codex was laid down. Which two of the following are the most useful additions to the Syndicate code if attempting to convey the following message?

Modern politicians need to use the internet, television and road tours to communicate effectively with their people.

A. Politician
B. Internet
C. Television
D. Road tours
E. Communicate

23. What's the best way to translate the following into Syndicate code?

To have and to hold,

from this day forward,

for better, for worse,

for richer, for poorer,

in sickness, and in health.

A. ❽,☗ (ᵭ,♐,✪ᵭ,❋ᵭ, ♦☀☞,☺ᵭ)

B. ❽,♌ (ᵭ,♐,✪ᵭ,❋ᵭ, ♦☀☞,☺ᵭ)

C. ♌☗ (ᵭ,♐,✪ᵭ,❋ᵭ, ♦☀☞,☺ᵭ)

D. ❽,♌☗ (ᵭ,♐,✪ᵭ,❋ᵭ, ♦☀☞,☺ᵭ)

E. ❽ (ᵭ,♐,✪ᵭ,❋ᵭ, ♦☀☞,☺ᵭ)

24. What's the best way to translate the following into Syndicate code?

    Whoever wants to be happy, let him be so: of tomorrow there's no knowing.

    A. ☺(☺♂),☖(♎♇)

    B. ☺(☺♂),♎(☖♇)

    C. ☺(☺♂),☖(♎,♎♇)

    D. ☺♂,☖(♎,♎♇)

    E. (☺☺)♂,☖♎♇

25. What's the best way to translate the following into syndicate code?

    The gold is hidden in the cardinal's palace.

    A. ⌂❖,♟✿

    B. ⌂❖,♟❖(✿✿)

    C. ♟⌂❖,✿✿

    D. ♟(✿✿),⌂

    E. ⌂❖,♟(✿✿)

26. What's the best way to translate the following into syndicate code?

    The knight charged on horseback into the satanic cult's fire.

    A. ♘,✗,♟🏛✝⌂⌂),♋

    B. ♘,✗☞,✝⌂⌂,♋

    C. ♘,✗☞,♟(✝⌂⌂),♋

    D. ♘,♉☞,♟(✝⌂⌂),♋

    E. ♘,✗☞,♟(✝⌂⌂),♋

27. What's the best interpretation of the following Penumbra message?

    ♎,✝,💣,🔔,♎,✝

    A. What if the cardinal killed the Pope?
    B. If the Pope dies, the cardinal will become Pope.
    C. If the Pope dies, the cardinalate will elect a new pope.
    D. The cardinal might be plotting to assassinate the Pope.
    E. The dead Pope would not have approved of the cardinal.

28. What's the best interpretation of the following Penumbra message?

    🔔,♒,✝,📖,✝

    A. The cardinal has an audience with the Pope.
    B. If the Pope dies, the cardinal will become Pope.
    C. The cardinal would like to speak to both popes.
    D. The cardinal sailed to Rome for an audience with the Pope.
    E. The old Pope sailed to Rome with the cardinal.

Situational Judgement Test

Mrs Jones is about to be discharged after a hip operation. Unfortunately, she has no friends or relatives who are able to care for her at home. Mr Digby, the consultant orthopaedic surgeon, suggests arranging some home help, but Mrs Jones is adamant that she does not want or need any help.

How **appropriate** are each of the following responses by **Mr Digby** in this situation?

1. Explore Mrs Jones's concerns about receiving home help.

   A. A very appropriate thing to do.

   B. Appropriate, but not ideal.

   C. Inappropriate, but not awful.

   D. A very inappropriate thing to do.

2. Explore possible alternatives to home help.

   A. A very appropriate thing to do.

   B. Appropriate, but not ideal.

   C. Inappropriate, but not awful.

   D. A very inappropriate thing to do.

3. Delay Mrs Jones's discharge until she is mobile enough to manage alone at home.

   A. A very appropriate thing to do.

   B. Appropriate, but not ideal.

   C. Inappropriate, but not awful.

   D. A very inappropriate thing to do.

4. Discharge Mrs Jones without any further ado, because she probably has the mental capacity to make this sort of decision.

   A. A very appropriate thing to do.

   B. Appropriate, but not ideal.

   C. Inappropriate, but not awful.

   D. A very inappropriate thing to do.

A psychiatrist and a social worker have arrived at the home of John Smith, a patient with acute schizophrenia. They have grounds to suspect that John's condition is deteriorating, and want to assess his mental state with a possible view to hospital admission. They knock on the door repeatedly, but no one answers.

How **appropriate** are each of the following responses by the **mental health team** in this situation?

5. Ask the neighbours whether they know John's whereabouts.

    A. A very appropriate thing to do.
    B. Appropriate, but not ideal.
    C. Inappropriate, but not awful.
    D. A very inappropriate thing to do.

6. Call John's nearest relative, who is very concerned about John, and ask where John may be.

    A. A very appropriate thing to do.
    B. Appropriate, but not ideal.
    C. Inappropriate, but not awful.
    D. A very inappropriate thing to do.

7. Call the police and ask them to force access to the property.

    A. A very appropriate thing to do.
    B. Appropriate, but not ideal.
    C. Inappropriate, but not awful.
    D. A very inappropriate thing to do.

8. Try to call John on his mobile number.

    A. A very appropriate thing to do.
    B. Appropriate, but not ideal.
    C. Inappropriate, but not awful.
    D. A very inappropriate thing to do.

9. Aim to return in one month's time.

    A. A very appropriate thing to do.
    B. Appropriate, but not ideal.
    C. Inappropriate, but not awful.
    D. A very inappropriate thing to do.

A psychiatrist and a social worker have arrived at the home of John Smith, a patient with acute schizophrenia. They have grounds to suspect that John's condition is deteriorating, and want to assess his mental state with a possible view to hospital admission. When they knock on the door, John keeps the door on the chain and angrily abuses and threatens them.

How **appropriate** are each of the following responses by the **mental health team** in this situation?

10. Insist that John opens the door and lets them in.

    A. A very appropriate thing to do.

    B. Appropriate, but not ideal.

    C. Inappropriate, but not awful.

    D. A very inappropriate thing to do.

11. Leave without delay.

    A. A very appropriate thing to do.

    B. Appropriate, but not ideal.

    C. Inappropriate, but not awful.

    D. A very inappropriate thing to do.

12. Return later with more people and security.

    A. A very appropriate thing to do.

    B. Appropriate, but not ideal.

    C. Inappropriate, but not awful.

    D. A very inappropriate thing to do.

Mrs Bridgens, a patient with a recent diagnosis of breast cancer, tells her GP that she is seeking to end her life.

How **important** to take into account are the following considerations for **the GP** when deciding how to respond to the situation?

13. The patient's degree of intent.

A. A very important.
B. Important.
C. Of minor importance.
D. Not important at all.

14. The patient's mental state.

A. A very important.
B. Important.
C. Of minor importance.
D. Not important at all.

15. The patient's level of social support.

A. A very important.
B. Important.
C. Of minor importance.
D. Not important at all.

16. The patient's likelihood of recovering from breast cancer.

A. A very important.
B. Important.
C. Of minor importance.
D. Not important at all.

Lucy Light, a patient who was hospitalised for a psychotic relapse in her bipolar disorder six months ago, asks Dr Beaufort, her psychiatrist, to reinstate her suspended driving licence.

How **important** to take into account are the following considerations for **Dr Beaufort** when deciding how to respond to the situation?

17. Lucy's current mental state.

    A. A very important.
    B. Important.
    C. Of minor importance.
    D. Not important at all.

18. Lucy's compliance with her medication.

    A. A very important.
    B. Important.
    C. Of minor importance.
    D. Not important at all.

19. The nature and degree of any medication side-effects that Lucy may be suffering from.

    A. A very important.
    B. Important.
    C. Of minor importance.
    D. Not important at all.

20. Lucy's need to drive.

    A. A very important.
    B. Important.
    C. Of minor importance.
    D. Not important at all.

Linda Sheffield is taken to A&E after injuring her leg in a serious road traffic accident. Dr Banerjee, a junior doctor in A&E, manages to stem the bleeding. Linda has lost a lot of blood and requires a blood transfusion. However, she is a Jehovah's Witness and makes it abundantly clear that she does not want a blood transfusion.

How **appropriate** are each of the following responses by **Dr Banerjee** in this situation?

21. Ensure that Linda is aware of the risks involved in her refusal.

A. A very appropriate thing to do.
B. Appropriate, but not ideal.
C. Inappropriate, but not awful.
D. A very inappropriate thing to do.

22. Discharge Linda, because there's nothing further that can be done for her.

A. A very appropriate thing to do.
B. Appropriate, but not ideal.
C. Inappropriate, but not awful.
D. A very inappropriate thing to do.

23. Challenge Linda's religious views.

A. A very appropriate thing to do.
B. Appropriate, but not ideal.
C. Inappropriate, but not awful.
D. A very inappropriate thing to do.

24. Seek advice from a senior colleague.

A. A very appropriate thing to do.
B. Appropriate, but not ideal.
C. Inappropriate, but not awful.
D. A very inappropriate thing to do.

James Sheffield, who is 10 years old, is taken to A&E after injuring his leg in a serious road traffic accident. Dr Banerjee, a junior doctor in A&E, manages to stem the bleeding. James has lost a lot of blood and requires a blood transfusion. However, his mother, Linda Sheffield, who is a Jehovah's Witness, refuses to consent to a blood transfusion.

How **appropriate** are each of the following responses by **Dr Banerjee** in this situation?

25. Withhold the blood transfusion.

    A. A very appropriate thing to do.

    B. Appropriate, but not ideal.

    C. Inappropriate, but not awful.

    D. A very inappropriate thing to do.

26. Immediately seek support from a senior colleague.

    A. A very appropriate thing to do.

    B. Appropriate, but not ideal.

    C. Inappropriate, but not awful.

    D. A very inappropriate thing to do.

27. Immediately seek advice from his defence body.

    A. A very appropriate thing to do.

    B. Appropriate, but not ideal.

    C. Inappropriate, but not awful.

    D. A very inappropriate thing to do.

Arun, a fourth-year medical student who is very familiar with the hospital, is running late to an appointment with his supervisor when a patient with a Zimmer frame hails him in the corridor and asks him for directions to the cardiology outpatients' clinic. Arun has already rescheduled the appointment with his supervisor twice, and is keen not to antagonise her any further.

How **appropriate** are each of the following responses by **Arun** in this situation?

28. Politely apologise to the patient and explain that he's in a hurry.

A. A very appropriate thing to do.
B. Appropriate, but not ideal.
C. Inappropriate, but not awful.
D. A very inappropriate thing to do.

29. Wave at the overhead signs and keep on walking.

A. A very appropriate thing to do.
B. Appropriate, but not ideal.
C. Inappropriate, but not awful.
D. A very inappropriate thing to do.

30. Give the patient careful directions and then excuse himself to his supervisor for being late.

A. A very appropriate thing to do.
B. Appropriate, but not ideal.
C. Inappropriate, but not awful.
D. A very inappropriate thing to do.

31. Ignore the patient, because someone else will be able to give directions.

A. A very appropriate thing to do.
B. Appropriate, but not ideal.
C. Inappropriate, but not awful.
D. A very inappropriate thing to do.

Tim is in the hospital lift with two fellow medical students who are naming and discussing several patients who have recently been admitted to the clinical decisions unit. There are eight other people in the lift.

How **appropriate** are each of the following responses by **Tim** in this situation?

32. Quietly warn his fellow medical students that they are breaking the confidentiality of their patients.

   A. A very appropriate thing to do.
   B. Appropriate, but not ideal.
   C. Inappropriate, but not awful.
   D. A very inappropriate thing to do.

33. Wait until they are out of the lift, and then have a word with his fellow medical students.

   A. A very appropriate thing to do.
   B. Appropriate, but not ideal.
   C. Inappropriate, but not awful.
   D. A very inappropriate thing to do.

34. Subtly change the subject of the conversation.

   A. A very appropriate thing to do.
   B. Appropriate, but not ideal.
   C. Inappropriate, but not awful.
   D. A very inappropriate thing to do.

35. Report the medical students to the senior tutor.

   A. A very appropriate thing to do.
   B. Appropriate, but not ideal.
   C. Inappropriate, but not awful.
   D. A very inappropriate thing to do.

36. Do nothing at all.

   A. A very appropriate thing to do.
   B. Appropriate, but not ideal.
   C. Inappropriate, but not awful.
   D. A very inappropriate thing to do.

Clarissa is a 20-year-old student who takes drugs and regularly partakes in casual, unprotected sexual intercourse. One day, she accidentally falls pregnant and then seeks to terminate her pregnancy. However, her GP, Dr Cosgrove, has strong Christian beliefs, and objects both to abortion and to Clarissa's dissolute lifestyle.

How **important** to take into account are the following considerations for **Dr Cosgrove** when deciding how to respond to the situation?

37. The need to treat Clarissa with respect.

A. A very important.
B. Important.
C. Of minor importance.
D. Not important at all.

38. Clarissa's entitlement to care and treatment.

A. A very important.
B. Important.
C. Of minor importance.
D. Not important at all.

39. The ideal of practising in accordance with her (Dr Cosgrove's) own beliefs.

A. A very important.
B. Important.
C. Of minor importance.
D. Not important at all.

40. The need to avoid causing Clarissa further distress.

A. A very important.
B. Important.
C. Of minor importance.
D. Not important at all.

Mrs Aloke is requesting a second breast augmentation from Mr Haridas, a cosmetic surgeon in private practice. However, Mr Haridas is concerned that the surgery may not have the desired outcome and that the risk of surgery could outweigh the benefit. Moreover, Mrs Aloke is adamant that Mr Haridas should not liaise with her GP, Dr Banning, who opposes the surgery.

How **important** to take into account are the following considerations for **Mr Haridas** when deciding how to respond to the situation?

41. Whether the proposed intervention is in the overall benefit of the patient.

A. A very important.
B. Important.
C. Of minor importance.
D. Not important at all.

42. The patient's request for the intervention.

A. A very important.
B. Important.
C. Of minor importance.
D. Not important at all.

43. The fact that the patient is paying for the procedure herself.

A. A very important.
B. Important.
C. Of minor importance.
D. Not important at all.

44. The need to have access to the patient's medical records.

A. A very important.
B. Important.
C. Of minor importance.
D. Not important at all.

The mother of 6-year-old Will is upset that he's being bullied at school because of his protruding ears. She asks Dr Alcock, their GP, to refer Will to a paediatric surgeon to have his ears pinned back. The following day, Will's father, who is divorced from Will's mother, rings Dr Alcock to say that he objects to the operation on the grounds that it's not in Will's best interests.

How **important** to take into account are the following considerations for **Dr Alcock** when deciding how to respond to the situation?

45. Will's best interests.

   A. A very important.

   B. Important.

   C. Of minor importance.

   D. Not important at all.

46. Will's views.

   A. A very important.

   B. Important.

   C. Of minor importance.

   D. Not important at all.

47. The fact that Will's parents are divorced.

   A. A very important.

   B. Important.

   C. Of minor importance.

   D. Not important at all.

48. The need for a third-party view, for example, from Will's teacher.

   A. A very important.

   B. Important.

   C. Of minor importance.

   D. Not important at all.

Mrs Chalmers is upset with her GP, Dr Feniband, after he promised to refer her to a gastroenterologist and then omitted to do so. Mrs Chalmers' symptoms have worsened, and she is threatening to file a complaint against Dr Feniband.

How **appropriate** are each of the following responses by **Dr Feniband** in this situation?

49. Apologise to Mrs Chalmers.

    A. A very appropriate thing to do.
    B. Appropriate, but not ideal.
    C. Inappropriate, but not awful.
    D. A very inappropriate thing to do.

50. Explain to Mrs Chalmers why he omitted to refer her.

    A. A very appropriate thing to do.
    B. Appropriate, but not ideal.
    C. Inappropriate, but not awful.
    D. A very inappropriate thing to do.

51. Unilaterally put an end to his professional relationship with Mrs Chalmers.

    A. A very appropriate thing to do.
    B. Appropriate, but not ideal.
    C. Inappropriate, but not awful.
    D. A very inappropriate thing to do.

52. Try, as far as possible, to put things right for Mrs Chalmers.

    A. A very appropriate thing to do.
    B. Appropriate, but not ideal.
    C. Inappropriate, but not awful.
    D. A very inappropriate thing to do.

53. Suggest to Mrs Chalmers that her behaviour is unreasonable.

    A. A very appropriate thing to do.
    B. Appropriate, but not ideal.
    C. Inappropriate, but not awful.
    D. A very inappropriate thing to do.

A young surgeon, Mr Fulford, has just been diagnosed with narcolepsy ('sleeping sickness') by his GP, Dr Vasanti. Mr Fulford occasionally suffers from sleep attacks, when he falls asleep suddenly and without warning. Dr Vasanti is worried about the implications for Mr Fulford's clinical practice.

How **important** to take into account are the following considerations for **Dr Vasanti** when deciding how to respond to the situation?

54. The severity of Mr Fulford's condition.

    A. A very important.
    B. Important.
    C. Of minor importance.
    D. Not important at all.

55. The type of work that Mr Fulford undertakes.

    A. A very important.
    B. Important.
    C. Of minor importance.
    D. Not important at all.

56. The safety of Mr Fulford's patients.

    A. A very important.
    B. Important.
    C. Of minor importance.
    D. Not important at all.

57. Mr Fulford's response to treatment.

    A. A very important.
    B. Important.
    C. Of minor importance.
    D. Not important at all.

58. Mr Fulford's opinion on the matter.

    A. A very important.
    B. Important.
    C. Of minor importance.
    D. Not important at all.

Dr Chan, a new registrar on a geriatric unit, is appalled to discover that some patients on the ward are not being given sufficient food or water. In one case, a patient wet her bed because no one was available to help her to the toilet.

How **appropriate** are each of the following responses by **Dr Chan** in this situation?

59. Do nothing, because nursing care is not his responsibility.

A. A very appropriate thing to do.
B. Appropriate, but not ideal.
C. Inappropriate, but not awful.
D. A very inappropriate thing to do.

60. Report the stroke unit to the national Care Quality Commission.

A. A very appropriate thing to do.
B. Appropriate, but not ideal.
C. Inappropriate, but not awful.
D. A very inappropriate thing to do.

61. Discuss the matter with his consultant.

A. A very appropriate thing to do.
B. Appropriate, but not ideal.
C. Inappropriate, but not awful.
D. A very inappropriate thing to do.

62. Discuss the matter with the nurse in charge.

A. A very appropriate thing to do.
B. Appropriate, but not ideal.
C. Inappropriate, but not awful.
D. A very inappropriate thing to do.

63. Put together a small multidisciplinary team to carry out an audit of basic care on the stroke unit.

A. A very appropriate thing to do.
B. Appropriate, but not ideal.
C. Inappropriate, but not awful.
D. A very inappropriate thing to do.

Foster is a 9-year-old boy who has recently been diagnosed with cancer. Foster's grandmother died of cancer last year, and his parents are reluctant to inform him of his diagnosis. However, Dr Shah, the consultant in charge of his care, feels that Foster ought to be told.

How **important** to take into account are the following considerations for **Dr Shah** when deciding how to respond to the situation?

64. Foster's parents' concerns about informing him of his diagnosis.

   A. A very important.
   B. Important.
   C. Of minor importance.
   D. Not important at all.

65. Foster's capacity to understand his diagnosis and its implications.

   A. A very important.
   B. Important.
   C. Of minor importance.
   D. Not important at all.

66. Foster's attitude to his illness.

   A. A very important.
   B. Important.
   C. Of minor importance.
   D. Not important at all.

67. The General Medical Council's guidance on this issue.

   A. A very important.
   B. Important.
   C. Of minor importance.
   D. Not important at all.

68. Foster's parents' wishes.

   A. A very important.
   B. Important.
   C. Of minor importance.
   D. Not important at all.

Nathan has recently been diagnosed with HIV/AIDS. He's currently having sexual relations with two different partners, but asks Dr Sharma not to tell them about his diagnosis. Dr Sharma isn't sure what to do.

How **important** to take into account are the following considerations for **Dr Sharma** when deciding how to respond to the situation?

69. Nathan's right to confidentiality.

    A. A very important.
    B. Important.
    C. Of minor importance.
    D. Not important at all.

70. Whether Nathan has had or intends to have unprotected sexual intercourse with his either of his partners.

    A. A very important.
    B. Important.
    C. Of minor importance.
    D. Not important at all.

71. The fact that Nathan has two partners.

    A. A very important.
    B. Important.
    C. Of minor importance.
    D. Not important at all.

Chapter 10

Practice Test One: Answers and Explanations

In This Chapter

▶ Answering the questions in Practice Test One

▶ Understanding the answers

Verbal Reasoning

1. A: True

   To the population of Rome, the corn monopoly 'was considered as the immediate cause' of the famine. The famine, alongside pestilence (disease), was one of the 'calamities of Rome' that led to the 'popular discontent' that culminated in the violent scenes of the passage. The passage describes a logical sequence starting with corn monopoly and ending with the violence.

   You don't need to know whether the corn monopoly was actually the cause of the famine in order to determine the statement's veracity – you simply need to know that the Romans considered it to be. The Romans may or may not have been correct.

2. A: True

   The passage describes Commodus as waking from a 'dream of pleasure' and being previously unconscious of the civil war. Therefore, Commodus was asleep when these events took place.

3. B: False

   The passage says that missiles thrown from houses on the streets checked the pursuit of the Praetorian cavalry. Therefore the crowd didn't retreat outside the city but fought the Praetorians from within the city.

A fatal ending

In reality, Commodus became increasingly megalomaniacal in the years that followed, including renaming Rome in his honour. Together with an economic and farming crisis, this behaviour led to his unpopularity and eventually to his assassination. Commodus was Emperor of Rome for as long as 12 years, which may surprise you if you know of him from the movie *Gladiator.* Commodus enjoyed competing in the gladiatorial arena, though doing so brought him more scorn from the Roman elite, who viewed this behaviour as scandalous.

4. C: Can't tell

The passage says only that Commodus 'might even yet have regained' the 'confidence of his subjects', not that he did so. You still don't know the actual outcome by the end of the passage.

5. C: Can't tell

The passage only says that the unfortunate 8-year-old was one of Oliver's early encounters, not the first person he met. The child may have been the first person or not, but you can't be certain from the passage. The complicating presence of the clause regarding *The New York Times,* between dashes in the relevant sentence of the passage, encourages careless eyes to miss the crucial qualifier.

6. C: Can't tell

The passage confirms that around half the population are obese. It says that these people have one of the highest incidences of heart disease and diabetes, but it doesn't say what that incidence is, so you can't tell whether the incidence is around half, higher or lower. Therefore, you can't prove or disprove the statement's truth based on the information in the passage.

Beware of statements that include one true fact and then tag on facts that you can't prove. Wrongly selecting 'True' as your answer here is easily done.

If the statement began with the phrase 'The passage says that . . .', the answer would be 'False' rather than 'Can't tell', because the statement would then be a specific case rather than a general statement.

7. A: True

The passage says that if the show does well in the US, it will be re-exported to the UK. Therefore, British viewers will be able to see the show.

8. A: True

The passage refers to a long tradition of UK reality shows being success-fully adapted for the US. Therefore, these formats can work well in the US.

9. B: False

Price is certainly a determinant of the sales of sausages, but other factors play a part, such as the development of own brands by the supermarkets (as mentioned in the third paragraph) and the need for differentiation (first paragraph), as well as the attraction of premium price products (second paragraph).

 Highly exclusionary ('only') or universal ('all') statements are often false. Read the passage carefully to determine whether the text really does support the statement.

10. A: True

The second paragraph states that promotional support was recommended by the sales department to protect listings with the major supermarkets.

11. A: True

The first paragraph states that 'profitability of the core sausage business had been in decline for five years, with the brand trapped in a vicious downward cycle of increasing price promotion, leading to less funds for marketing and innovation'. Thus, falling profits mean less money for marketing.

12. A: True

Sales dropped from 35 per cent to 19 per cent between 1999 and 2006.

13. C: Can't tell

Although the passage confirms that both shows were prime-time music programmes, the two shows don't necessarily attract the same audience demographic.

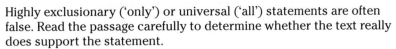

Polarising profits

The sausage firm featured in the excerpt is fic-tional, but the dilemma faced by the company is real. Operating as an undifferentiated mass-market retailer is increasingly hard. Sales are increasingly driven either to low-cost budget brands or to high-end, highly differentiated elite products. The middle market needs to focus on getting across what makes it unique in order to maintain margins and avoid entering an unwin-nable price war against low-cost brands.

14. A: True

The passage confirms that Syco TV makes both *X Factor* and *Britain's Got Talent,* and that Syco TV is Cowell's. Thus, Cowell has a financial interest in both shows.

15. C: Can't tell

Based on the information in the passage, you can't tell which partner makes more money.

16. B: False

The article confirms, in different places, that both Syco TV and Syco Music are at least partly Cowell's.

17. B: Foolishness

The passage says that the second man, who is deemed to be the more courageous, cannot in fact be the more courageous, because his behaviour is more foolish than that of the first man, 'and foolish behaviour is both disgraceful and harmful, whereas courage is always a fine and noble thing.'

In the third sentence, fear (A) is spoken of as the subject matter of courage, so it's a synonym more than an antonym.

In the fourth sentence, courage is compared to recklessness (C) (but not opposed to it) and equated with knowledge (D).

18. B: Courage is always a fine and noble thing.

The assumption that courage is always a fine and noble thing is used to demonstrate that the second man, whose behaviour is more foolish and therefore the opposite of fine and noble, isn't in fact the more courageous.

Although the author clearly thinks that most people have a mistaken notion of courage, he doesn't assume that whatever people think must be wrong (A).

The author does assume that children and animals have no sense, but this isn't central to his arguments (C).

The example from Homer merely 'suggests' (rather than 'proves' or 'demonstrates') that courage amounts not to blind recklessness (D).

19. D: Other virtues such as patience and moderation also amount to knowledge.

This is a tricky question owing to the use of a negative in the stem and another negative in one of the options. Just remember that two negatives make a positive!

The passage clearly states that courage amounts to knowledge, so A can definitely be inferred. The second paragraph states that 'fear is produced by anticipated evil things, but not by evil things that have happened or that are happening', from which it can be inferred that you can't fear things that are in the past (B). The text also states that 'for any science of knowledge, there is not one science of the past, one of the present, and one of the future', from which it can be inferred that the principles of science or knowledge don't change with time (C).

However probable it may seem that other virtues such as patience and moderation also amount to knowledge, there's nothing in the passage to suggest this.

20. C: Popular opinion is usually a good guide to the truth.

The passage states that most people seem to think that courage amounts to blind recklessness, suggesting that, while the author believes that people take words and concepts for granted (A), he doesn't believe that popular opinion is usually a good guide to the truth (C).

The author often analyses the way that words are used to make his arguments, and would certainly agree that 'careful analysis of the way that words are used can help us to clarify concepts' (B). As for D, it's simply a rephrasing or interpretation of the author's conclusion.

21. A: True

The author compares the town of Harper's Ferry favourably with Lucerne. You can logically say that the author finds the town more beautiful.

22. A: True

The passage is quite flowery but it does state that the town is faced on at least two sides by the Shenandoah River and the Potomac River, and that you can find it 'nestling inside' the confluence (joining point) of these two rivers.

23. C: Can't tell

Captain Brown believed this statement to be true, but the passage doesn't provide the information required for you to say whether it is true. In reality, the slave population remained surprisingly loyal even during the Civil War itself, but how much of this loyalty was down to habit or fear – rather than satisfaction with arrangements at the time – is uncertain.

24. B: False

The passage says that after securing the arsenal and armoury, Brown planned to return to the mountainous regions of the area to rally slave support. Therefore, he didn't intend to make a stand in the town.

25. B: False

She only 'wished' something wonderful would happen. Although she doesn't know whether something wonderful will or will not happen, the answer to the statement isn't 'Can't tell', because her uncertainty is opposed to the statement. The answer is therefore 'False'.

26. C: Can't tell

The passage goes to great lengths to tell us that the old gentlemen spoke to every passenger in turn – but to preserve story surprise the passage doesn't tell you what the gentlemen actually said to the passengers. Even with the benefit of the hindsight granted by the rest of the passage, you still don't know whether his request was limited to the passengers all reading the requested article in the newspaper (which was then followed by a spontaneous and contagious waving by the passengers on passing the children), or whether the waving was included in his request. After you read the article, assuming that the waving is prearranged is easy – but you cannot conclude this from the evidence in the passage.

27. A: True

The passage states that the children had given their love to the train freely for a long time before the events of the passage.

28. C: Can't tell

You can't be certain of what the three children knew was going to happen. You can say that Bobbie didn't expect it to happen, because in the first sentence she wished for something unexpectedly wonderful to happen. But you can't tell what the other two children knew, or didn't know, about the events of that day and their cause. Without spoiling the ending of *The Railway Children,* we can safely reveal that in the novel none of the children expected or understood the happy reason for the waving – but they soon would.

29. A: True

The passage describes social media as 'a term that encompasses the transactional, search and marketing components of social media'. This description is logically equivalent to being a descriptive term for how social media interacts with business.

30. C: Can't tell

Although the passage says that younger generations of people were the first to adopt Facebook, the text doesn't provide any reasons for this early adoption. The reason may be that younger people are less socially inhibited, but equally the reason may be that younger people have less experience in understanding how maintaining definite boundaries of social interaction can be helpful. Or maybe the effect is random and no reason exists. More prosaically, the reason may be that Facebook was originally restricted to college students, and so most older people were unable to sign up, giving Facebook cachet among younger groups.

31. C: Can't tell

The passage describes status updates as being at least partially an outlet for bragging. The passage also describes functions other than updating your status. The passage doesn't indicate how common bragging is relative to other updates – and of course, status updates aren't the entirety of sharing on social media.

32. A: True

The passage quotes a Nielsen study suggesting that 78 per cent of people trust their peers' opinions. Whether they're wise to do so is another matter.

33. C: Can't tell

The passage essentially says that water scarcity will be an increasingly difficult problem for China to manage, but it doesn't say that China will be unable to manage it.

34. C: Can't tell

The passage tells you that China has 8 per cent of the world's fresh water, and that China has less water than it needs by international standards, but the passage doesn't mention what percentage of its water needs China can meet.

35. A: True

The article unequivocally states that China has less than a quarter of the world average in terms of per capita availability of water reserves. It also states that 'China will be under severe water stress, as defined by the international standard'. By combining this information with the earlier sentence that states that China has widespread problems of water scarcity, you can deduce that China already has less water than it needs by international standards.

36. A: True

The article states that half of China's wheat and corn grows on the North China Plain, and also that the area has extensive peach orchards. This information is enough to classify the area as a major agricultural centre – you don't need to know *how* major (and indeed you can't work out how major from the text).

37. C: Can't tell

You know only that a small group of Canadian researchers were interested enough in zombies to model an outbreak. You've no information on what the rest of the Canadian research community thought about it, although we can guess that they may have chuckled . . .

38. B: False

You can remove – kill – zombies by pursuing the rather graphic procedure described in the passage.

39. A: True

The study demonstrated that a city of half a million people can be overwhelmed within four days.

40. B: False

    The study called for frequent and increasingly forceful attacks to eradicate the zombie threat. Thus, superior firepower can defeat zombies.

41. D: It isn't double the size of the old altar.

    Answers B and C are factually inaccurate, since the new altar is eight times (not four times) the volume of the original one and four times (not eight times) too big.

    Answers A and D are both correct, but answer D *best* summarises the potential problem, since it's written in the same terms as the oracular pronouncement which advised the Delians to *double the size* of their altar to Apollo.

42. A: Build an altar that is only approximately twice the volume of the first.

    Plato didn't advise the Delians to build an altar that's only approximately twice the volume of the first.

    However, the text clearly says that the Delians 'might take up the study of mathematics and philosophy so as to moderate their passions' (D). 'Failing that, they could always try building a third altar identical to the first and setting it beside the first or on top of it' (B, C).

43. B: The Delians thought that Plato might take their problem seriously.

    The Delians wouldn't have asked Plato for advice if they hadn't thought that he might take their problem seriously.

    Plato's reply to the Delians may well be tongue in cheek, or partly tongue in cheek, but it's impossible to be sure (A). Even if the Delians had known the method for doubling the volume of a cube, it's by no means certain that their feuding would have come to an end. That is simply what they believed (C). The method for doubling the volume of a cube has since been discovered, but it's impossible to infer this from the text (D).

44. D: Even before writing to Plato, the Delians understood in what way they had misinterpreted the oracular pronouncement.

    The Delians clearly had faith in the Delphic oracle or they would not have gone through so much trouble (A). Neither would they have written to Plato if they hadn't valued his opinion (B). Plato's reply clearly demonstrates that he understood the principles of geometry, and he's even aware that no one knows the method for doubling the volume of a cube (C).

    It's possible that the Delians understood in what way they'd misinterpreted the oracular pronouncement, but their attempt at doubling the size of their altar to Apollo together with their impulse to seek advice from abroad suggests that they didn't.

Quantitative Reasoning

1. C: 25%

   Four large caps and one mega-cap are present, making five companies at least large cap in size. Because the selection under consideration includes 20 companies, the percentage is $(5 \div 20) \times 100 = 25\%$.

2. B: 1:1

   Four large caps and four micro-caps are present, so the ratio is 4:4 = 1:1.

3. D: 10.5%

   The merger of two large caps to form a mega-cap means that there are now two mega-caps. However, the total number of companies falls from 20 to 19, as a result of the merger. The new percentage of mega-caps is therefore $(2 \div 19) \times 100 = 10.5\%$ (approximately).

4. E: 229

   The current market cap in sterling is 165 billion $\times$ 0.85 = 140.25 billion. Converting to US dollars gives $140.25 \times 1.63 = 228.6075$ billion = $229 billion (approximately).

5. B: 62%

   In total, 103 fatalities have occurred, and 64 up to the end of June, so the percentage is $(64 \div 103) \times 100 = 62\%$ to the nearest whole number.

6. A: 1.64

   You already know that of 103 total fatalities, 64 took place in the first half of the year, which means that $103 - 64 = 39$ fatalities occurred in the second half of the year. To find out how many times greater were your chances of dying in the first half compared with the second half, you divide one by the other:

   $64 \div 39 = 1.64$ to two decimal places.

7. D: 8.6

   You calculate the mean by dividing the total by the number of categories. In this case, you divide $103 \div 12 = 8.6$ to one decimal place.

8. D: 567%

   The modal average is the number that occurs most frequently, in this case 3 fatalities, which occurred in April, November and December. The deadliest month was June, with 20 fatalities – 17 more deaths than the mode. Expressed as a percentage:

   $(17 \div 3) \times 100 = 567\%$ to the nearest whole number.

9. E: No – his table is correct

For this question, you need to replicate the work that John put into drawing up his table. If you do so, you find that his table is correct.

10. B: 6

Four clubs will move up to the Football Royalty group (Man U, Man City, Newcastle, Sunderland) and one club will move up into the Aristocrats (Wolves). Given the current starting point of nine clubs in the Aristocrats, the net change of –3 will leave the Aristocrats with six clubs (Chelsea, Bolton, West Brom, Blackburn, Spurs, Wolves).

An alternate solution is to note that, to achieve the Aristocrats grouping in Table 8-4, teams need between 70 and 89 seasons in the top flight. If ten seasons are added to each value, the future Aristocrats will have current rankings of 60–79. According to Table 8-3, six teams are within these margins.

11. C: 101

This question demands a fairly straightforward calculation. The four Football Royalty clubs of Everton, Aston Villa, Liverpool and Arsenal have 109, 101, 97 and 95 seasons respectively, making a total of 402 seasons between them.

$402 \div 4 = 100.5$, which you round up to 101 to the nearest whole season.

12. D: 15

Wigan Athletic currently has 7 years in the top flight and needs a total of 20 years to become Bourgeoisie – that is, an extra 13 years. However, if Wigan is relegated twice and takes a year each time to return to the Premiership, the total number of years required is 15.

13. A: 331

You simply need to find the eighth highest score in the table, which is 331.

14. E: 674

The range is the difference between the highest and lowest figures in the sample. In this case, the range is $803 - 129 = 674$.

15. C: 55%

A cut-off score of 295 allows 11 players to qualify. As a percentage, this is $(11 \div 20) \times 100 = 55\%$.

16. D: 89%

The current average score of the bottom five players is $(129 + 141 + 163 + 164 + 184) \div 5 = 156.2$.

To reach a score of 295, the average score has to increase by $(295 - 156.2) = 138.8$ points. Expressed as a percentage of the current average, this is $138.8 \div 156.2 \times 100 = 89\%$ to the nearest whole percentage point.

Note that this represents an increase *of* 189% on the current average, but an increase *by* 89%.

You can quickly analyse this type of data display by ranking the data values relative to one another vertically on your portable white board. A quick glance shows you'll be going from 100 to 800. The first entry, 331, should go about one-third of the way down the page. The next entry of 803 should go towards the bottom. The entry 164 should be placed near the top; 330 should go immediately above 331 with no extra space for new entries . . . and so on. After all items of data are placed in order, the first three questions are simple to answer.

17. B: 114

The Radical SR8 LM takes 6 minutes 48 seconds (= 408 seconds) to do 20.6 km. You calculate speed by dividing the distance travelled by the time taken, but you also need to convert the units into miles and hours to calculate miles per hour (mph).

$(20.6 \div 1.6) \div (408 \div 3,600) = (20.6 \times 3,600) \div (1.6 \times 408) = 113.6$ (approximately) = 114 mph to the nearest whole number.

18. B: 7:24

The Zonda takes 33:04 to complete three laps, but 652 seconds of this time is wasted time. Without this wasted time, the Zonda would have taken $[(33 \times 60) + 4] - 652 = 1,332$ seconds to complete three laps. This is $1,332 \div 3 = 444$ seconds per lap.

Converting to minutes, you get $444 \div 60 = 7.4$ minutes or 7:24.

19. A: 365 hp

This answer is a simple ratio:

$680 \div 1210 \times 650 = 365$ hp (approximately).

20. C: 117 mph

This question isn't difficult, but the large number of calculations with many different units involved increases your chances of making an error. A survey of the units in the answer choices tells you that you need to choose km/h or mph for your calculation and convert to the other system if your answer doesn't match.

Lap 1: 120 mph = $120 \times 1.6 = 192$ km/h

Lap 2: 7:23 for 20.6 km = 443 seconds for 20.6 km = $20.6 \div (443 \div 3,600) = 167.40$ km/h to the nearest hundredth

Lap 3: $192 \times 105 \div 100 = 201.6$ km/h

Average speed = $(192 + 167.40 + 201.6) \div 3 = 187$ km/h

This figure doesn't match any of the km/h answer choices, so you need to convert to mph and hope for the best!

Converting to mph gives you $187 \div 1.6 = 116.88$ (approximately), which rounds to 117 mph.

21. E: 5.27:1

    The ratio is $52.7:(3 + 5.2 + 1.8) = 52.7:10 = 5.27:1$

22. C: The English make up a greater proportion of the total population in 2031 than in 2011.

    You can derive this answer by working through each proposition in turn. The English make up about 84 per cent of the population in 2011 and about 85 per cent in 2031, which is a greater proportion.

23. B: 13.4%

    Population in 2011 = $(52.7 + 3 + 5.2 + 1.8) = 62.7$ million

    Population in 2031 = $(60.4 + 3.3 + 5.4 + 2) = 71.1$ million

    Population increase = $71.1 - 62.7 = 8.4$ million

    The percentage increase is $8.4 \div 62.7 \times 100 = 13.4\%$ (approximately).

24. D: 57.4

    The range is the difference between the maximum and minimum values of the data – in this case, the maximum is the English population (60.4 million in 2031) and the minimum is the Welsh population (3 million in 2006). The difference is $(60.4 - 3) = 57.4$ million.

25. C: £7,010

    Each pair of Northampton Classics lasts 20 years. James will have a 40-year career, so he needs two pairs of each of the three types of shoe he wants to buy, making a total requirement of six pairs. The shoe cost is therefore $£650 \times 6 = £3,900$.

    He needs to resole each pair three times during its 20-year lifespan, giving a total of $6 \times 3 = 18$ resoles. The resoling cost is $£120 \times 18 = £2,160$.

    The polish costs are $£20 \times 40$ years = $£800$.

    James needs only three pairs of shoe trees, because he can reuse them. Tree costs are $£50 \times 3 = £150$.

    The total cost for wearing Northampton Classics over 40 years is therefore $(£3,900 + £2,160 + £800 + £150) = £7,010$.

26. E: £4,760

    James needs 20 pairs of each type of shoe, making a total of $20 \times 3 = 60$ pairs. The total shoe cost is therefore $60 \times £75 = £4,500$.

The shoe polish costs are £5 × 40 = £200. James needs six pairs of shoe trees, because they last only 20 years, making a total tree cost of 6 × £10 = £60

The total cost of wearing Mass Market shoes is therefore (£4,500 + £200 + £60) = £4,760.

27. E: The annual cost of wearing Mass Market shoes is £110.

This figure is false. The actual cost is £4,760 ÷ 40 = £119. All the other statements are true.

28. D: 26.7

The new resoling interval is proportionally increased to (4 ÷ 3) × 5 years = 6.67 years.

James can still resole each pair of shoes three times, meaning that the shoes now last 6.67 + (6.67 × 3) = 26.7 years (approximately).

Alternatively, you can simply multiply the initial 20-year lifespan figure by 4 and divide by 3.

29. C: 2:1

The odds of a variable mortgage holder increasing expenditure are 133 ÷ 52 (the number of variable mortgage holders who increased expenditure divided by the number of variable mortgage holders who didn't increase expenditure).

The odds of a non-mortgage holder increasing expenditure are 111 ÷ 89 (the number of non-mortgage holders who increased expenditure divided by the number of non-mortgage holders who didn't increase expenditure).

To calculate how much more likely the holder will be to increase expenditure compared with the non-holder, you compare 133 ÷ 52 with 111 ÷ 89:

(133 ÷ 52) ÷ (111 ÷ 89) = 2.56 ÷ 1.25 = 2.05 = 2:1 (approximately)

You can't simply compare the raw figures of 133:111, because the total number of people in each group differs – so you're not comparing like with like. You need to figure out the odds within each group and then compare the two odds with each other to find the overall odds.

Worth it or not?

You can see from the calculations in answers 25–28 that James needs to decide whether to spend an extra £56.25 per year to wear Northampton classics, based on any extra pleasure he will derive from the purchase of a more beautiful artisanal product. This annual difference is relatively small compared with the vast difference in upfront shoe purchase price. Although the manufacturers' names are fictional, the figures and assumptions in this question are realistic.

Medical statistics I

Statisticians call the calculation in answer 29 the odds ratio. Odds ratios occur frequently in medical and scientific papers when the authors want to judge whether a treatment (for example, a new antibiotic) has a benefit compared with either an old treatment or no treatment at all (for example, a placebo).

30. D: 72%

   133 increased out of a total of $(52 + 133) = 185$. The percentage is therefore $(133 \div 185) \times 100 = 72\%$ to the nearest whole per cent.

31. A: 0.16

   The proportion of people who increased expenditure by at least 10 per cent and who were variable mortgage holders is $133 \div (53 + 133) = 0.72$ (approximately). (This calculation is the same as in answer 30, but without converting the answer into a percentage.)

   The proportion of people increasing expenditure in the non-mortgage group is $111 \div (111 + 89) = 0.56$ (approximately). The difference is $(0.72 - 0.56) = 0.16$.

32. B: 23.1%

   The study has a total of 385, of whom 89 meet the criteria. The percentage likelihood ('chance') of randomly picking one of these people is therefore $(89 \div 385) \times 100 = 23.1\%$ (approximately).

Medical statistics II

Statisticians describe the calculation in answer 31 as the (absolute) risk difference. If, instead of comparing expenditure levels in groups with and without variable rate mortgages, you compare health outcomes in groups of sick people taking and not taking a new drug, you can invert the risk difference to calculate the number needed to treat (NNT) – that is, the number of people you need to give the new drug to in order to successfully treat one person.

In the mortgage example, the NNT doesn't mean much, but if you describe it in words you can say 'the number of people without variable mortgages who need to switch to variable mortgages in order that one extra person will be influenced enough by the interest rate cut to increase expenditure by at least 10 per cent'.

33. B: 1,550 m²

    This calculation is relatively simple:

    Wall surface area = $2(50 \times 2) + 2(25 \times 2) = 300$ m²

    Bottom surface area = $50 \times 25 = 1{,}250$ m²

    Total internal surface area = $300 + 1{,}250 = 1{,}550$ m²

34. D: 162,600

    This question requires careful thought and calculation. The internal surface area is 1,550 square metres. Each tile measures 10 cm × 10 cm, or 0.1 m × 0.1 m. The internal surface area therefore requires 1,550 ÷ $(0.1 \times 0.1) = 155{,}000$ tiles.

    You also need to calculate the border. You can break down the border into two rectangles that measure $[(50 + 0.5 + 0.5) \times 0.5]$ and two rectangles that measure (25×0.5).

    Alternatively you can break down the border into two rectangles that measure (50×0.5), two rectangles that measure (25×0.5) and four corner squares that measure (0.5×0.5).

    The total area of the border is 76 square metres.

    Because each tile measures 0.1 m × 0.1 m, the border needs $[76 \div (0.1 \times 0.1] = 7{,}600$ tiles. Adding that to the number of tiles for the internal surface area gives $155{,}000 + 7{,}600 = 162{,}600$.

35. C: £25,590

    The total number of tiles is 162,600, of which 2,500 are dark blue and 7,500 are non-slip, leaving 152,600 pale blue. The cost is therefore:

    $(152{,}600 \times 0.15) + (2{,}500 \times 0.18) + (7{,}500 \times 0.3) = 22{,}890 + 450 + 2{,}250 = £25{,}590$

36. B: The 170th day

    You have 162,600 tiles at 5 minutes per tile = 813, 000 minutes = 13,550 hours of work. Ten tilers working simultaneously each need to do $13{,}550 \div 10 = 1{,}355$ hours of work.

    Each tiler works eight hours a day, so the team takes $1{,}355 \div 8 = 169.37$ days.

    However, the tilers complete the job not on the 169th day but on the 170th day, because any fraction above a whole number of days pushes the job into the following day. The normal practice of rounding down when the figure after the decimal point is less than 5 doesn't apply here.

Abstract Reasoning

1, Set A; **2**, Set B; **3**, neither set; **4**, Set B; **5**, neither set

Explanation

All the shapes in Set A have curved edges. All the shapes in Set B have straight edges. The size, colour and orientation of the shapes demonstrate no commonality within the sets.

Test shape 1 contains only shapes with curved edges and therefore falls into Set A. Test shapes 2 and 4 contain only shapes with straight edges and so fall into Set B. Test shapes 3 and 5 contain shapes with both curved and straight edges and therefore don't fall into either set.

6, Set B; **7**, Set A; **8**, neither set; **9**, Set B; **10**, Set A

Explanation

All the objects in Set A have solid outer edges and no interruptions in any edges. All the objects in Set B have outer edges with interruptions regardless of the inner edges. The exact nature of the overall shape, the colour and the orientation show no consistent features of commonality.

Test shapes 7 and 10 have only objects with solid uninterrupted outer edges and so fall within Set A. Test shapes 6 and 9 have interrupted outlines and so fall in Set B. Test shape 8 contains objects with both solid and interrupted outlines and so falls into neither set.

11, neither set; **12**, neither set; **13**, Set B; **14**, neither set; **15**, Set B

Explanation

All members of both sets contain exactly one large shape and one or two smaller shapes.

All the examples in Set A contain a large shape that's internally replicated in the same colour. For instance, the top-left item contains a large white triangle with a smaller white inner triangle, and the top-right item contains a large white hexagon with a smaller white inner hexagon.

All the examples in Set B contain a large shape that's internally replicated in the opposite colour. For instance, the top-left item contains a large triangle with a smaller black inner triangle, and the top-right item contains a large white circle with a smaller black inner circle within it.

The placement and orientation of the large object within the box are irrelevant, and any small shapes featured in each item show no consistent features of commonality.

Test shapes 13 and 15 have large objects that are internally replicated with smaller black objects, and so fit in Set B. Test shape 12 contains a large object that's replicated internally by a smaller white item, but because it has a second large shape it goes into neither set. Test shape 11 has both types of internal replication and so falls into neither set. Test shape 14 has no internal replication whatsoever and so falls into neither set.

16, A; **17**, B

Explanation

In Set A, the number of angles in the shape corresponds to the number of *up* arrows *plus* one. In Set B, the number of angles in the shape corresponds to the number of *down* arrows *minus* one.

18, D

Explanation

The small shape on top becomes more elongated and switches colour. Meanwhile the bottom shape rotates by 180 degrees.

19, B

Explanation

The shapes rotate by 90 degrees clockwise. The circle on the triangle moves clockwise to the next point on the triangle. The circle in the square moves clockwise into the next corner of the square.

20, D

Explanation

The triangle in the top left corner rotates by 90 degrees clockwise each time. The number of small shapes goes up by one each time. Whether the small shapes are triangles, squares or circles is immaterial.

21, Set A; **22**, neither set; **23**, neither set; **24**, Set A; **25**, neither set

Explanation

All of Set A's objects have three borders, and all of Set B's objects have four borders.

Test shapes 21 and 24 contain only three-sided objects and so are in Set A. Test shapes 22, 23 and 25 contain objects with varying numbers of sides and so fall into neither set.

26, Set A; **27**, Set A; **28**, Set A; **29**, neither set; **30**, Set B

Explanation

Set A's objects are undivided. Set B's objects are subdivided.

Test shapes 26, 27 and 28 contain objects without subdivision, and so belong in Set A. Test shape 30 has subdivided objects, and so is part of Set B. Test shape 29 has a mixture of whole and divided objects and so isn't in Set A or Set B.

31, neither set; **32**, Set B; **33**, neither set; **34**, Set B; **35**, Set A

Explanation

The shapes in Set A overlap only once, whereas the shapes in Set B overlap twice.

Test shape 35 has only one area of overlap, and so is in Set A. Test shapes 32 and 34 have two overlapping areas, and so belong to Set B. Test shape 31 has no overlaps and test shape 33 has three overlaps, and so both fall into neither set.

36, Set B; **37**, neither set; **38**, Set A; **39**, Set B; **40**, Set A

Explanation

You can draw every shape in Set A continuously without lifting your pen from the paper or backtracking. To draw Set B's shapes, you need to lift the pen at least once or backtrack.

Test shapes 38 and 40 fit in Set A. Test shapes 36 and 39 are part of Set B. Test shape 37 contains one element that you can draw without lifting your pen; but it also contains one element that you can't draw without lifting your pen, and so fits in neither set.

Note that some people may argue that test shape 37 belongs to Set B on the basis that drawing the shapes in Set B require you to lift your pen at least once.

The reason this line of argument is incorrect is that the bottom-left shape in Set A also contains multiple elements. All this shape's component elements can be drawn without lifting. This fact allows you to postulate a rule that in cases where a shape has multiple elements, all those component elements must follow the overall rule of the shape. Test shape 37 has one element that follows the rule of Set A, and another element that follows Set B's rule, and this confirms it's in neither set.

41, A

Explanation

For each row, the signs move one along, with the right-most sign becoming the left-most sign.

42, A

Explanation

The sequence is a shape with at least one right angle, followed by a shape without right angles, followed by a shape with at least one right angle, and so on.

43, C

Explanation

The line of triangles is rotating by 45 degrees anticlockwise each time. At the same time, the first and fourth triangles are rotating 90 degrees anticlockwise each time. The second triangle always points down. The third triangle always points right.

44, C

Explanation

The outer shape changes from a circle to a square. The number of points at which the inner shape touches the border of the outer shape increases by one each time.

45, A

Explanation

The superimposed shapes shift in order. The outermost becomes the innermost and the innermost becomes the outermost.

46, Set A; **47**, neither set; **48**, Set B; **49**, neither set; **50**, neither set

Explanation

The black circle is the key to these sets. In Set A, if the black circle is at the top of the shape, the arrow points up. If the black circle is in the middle, the arrow is horizontal. If the black circle is at the bottom, the arrow points down. In Set B, the top/bottom rule is reversed but the middle rule remains the same.

Test shape 46 obeys Set A's rules. Test shape 48 obeys Set B's rules. Test shape 47 has no black circle and so belongs to neither set. Test shapes 49 and 50 belong neither to Set A nor to Set B as the circles and arrows follow neither set of rules.

51, A; **52**, A

Explanation

In Set A, the circle's always above the square. In Set B, the square's always above the circle.

53, D; **54**, C

Explanation

In Set A, an area of intersection – if any – is always coloured black. In Set B, an area of intersection – if any – is always white.

55, B

Explanation

The line switches from horizontal to vertical and then back to horizontal. The two shapes at either end are always the same.

Decision Analysis

1. A: The cardinal will kill the king.

   🔔, ⏳💣, ᧞

   = Cardinal, Then Kill, King

   = Cardinal, kill at some point in the future, king = The cardinal will kill the king

   You can't express the future perfect tense using the Turin codex, but this answer is as close as you can get. No other option fits the code anyway.

2. C: The queen will persuade the king to pay us.

   ♍, ⏳📖, ᧞, ✉, (⚫●)

   = Queen, Then Talk, King, Pay (I you)

   = The queen will talk to the king to pay us

   = The queen will persuade the king to pay us

3. B: The Pope rides to meet his cardinals.

   ✝, ⚹, 🔔🔔

   = Pope, Ride, Cardinal Cardinal

   = The Pope rides cardinals

   = The Pope rides to meet his cardinals

   Without reading the options, you may leave the translation as 'The Pope rides cardinals', although this phrase doesn't sound terribly dignified . . .

4. D: The knights won't fight us today.

   🏴🏴, ♌👃

   = Knight Knight, Now Cowardly

   = Knights, are now cowardly

   = The knights won't fight us today

   You can encode this message in other ways, but only this choice from the list of options is a plausible decoding.

5. A: The queen is furious at the king's rapid retreat from battle.

♏, ☹, ᧿, ☞ 🖐, ☹(💣💥💣💥)

= Queen, Angry, King, Quickly Cowardly, Angry (Kill Kill)

= Queen is angry with king, rapid retreat from site of violent killings

= The queen is furious at the king's rapid retreat from battle

6. A: ✉, ✞, ☹📖, ᧿

= Pay, Pope, Angry Talk, King

= Bribe the Pope to talk angrily to the king

= Bribe the Pope to defy the king

The other options don't translate correctly to the English phrase in the question. Option B is Pope, Angry Talk, Pay King. This option may mean that the Pope is defying the king, but the pairing of the symbols of pay and king together most plausibly translate to the king being paid something (maybe taxes).

Option C mentions a knight, which isn't in the English phrase. Option D invokes killing as well as defiant talk, and doesn't mention the Pope, so is a worse translation. Option E includes the Pope, but also includes killing; the late placement of the symbol for Pope suggests that both the Pope and the king are being killed and angrily spoken to.

7. D: The peasants may not choose to take your bribe.

💧💧, ♎(🎱🖐), ●✉

= Peasant Peasant, Conditional (Take Negative), You Pay

= Peasants, may not take, your payment

= The peasants may not choose to take your bribe

You can quickly eliminate some of the other answers by comparing what symbols are present in the options. The English phrase talks about choosing, but several options include the symbols for 'angry' or 'kill'. These can be rapidly excluded as possible answers.

8. E: Rich knights will remain loyal to the king.

✡(⌐ ⌐), ⧗☺, ⌐

= Rich (Knight Knight), Then Calm, King

= Rich knights will stay calm, king

= Rich knights will remain loyal to the king

9. A: The Pope calmly ordered the execution of the rebel cardinal by burning at the stake.

✝, ☺📖, 🔥, 🔔, ♋

= Pope, Calm Talk, Kill, Negative Cardinal, Burn

= The Pope calmly ordered the execution of the bad cardinal by burning

= The Pope calmly ordered the execution of the rebel cardinal by burning at the stake

Despite the absence of any code for 'stake', this answer is the best-fit (or least-worst) option from the choices available.

The roles of the Pope and the cardinal are reversed in option B. Option C is wrong because the code has the symbol for calm, but the Pope in option C is furious, implying a greater degree of agitation. Option D has the cardinals (plural), but there is no indication in the code of more than one cardinal. Option E is wrong because, like option C, it has a more animated pope than implied by the use of the symbol for calm.

10. C: The peasants fought bravely to defend their homes from the evil knights.

🔴🔴, 💧☹, ☺(❖ ❖), ♟(⌐ ⌐)

= Peasant, Peasant, Brave Angry, Calm (Home Home), Negative (Knight Knight)

= The peasants, bravely angry to keep calm homes from bad knights

= The peasants fought bravely to defend their homes from the evil knights

11. D: I'll pay you to sail to Ravenna and kill the cardinal there.

○ ✉, ● 〰, Ravenna, ⌛ 🩸☄, 🔔

= I Pay, You Sail, Ravenna, Then Kill, Cardinal

= I pay you to sail to Ravenna and then kill the cardinal

= I'll pay you to sail to Ravenna and kill the cardinal there

12. C: We subdue both king and Pope.

(○ ●)☺(∿ ✝)

= (I You) Calm (King Pope)

= We subdue both king and Pope

13. B: The knight and his squire fight bravely.

⚑ 🩸, ☝(☹ 🩸☄)

= Knight Peasant, Positive (Angry Kill)

= The knight and peasant fight well

= The knight and his squire fight bravely

14. E: The King ordered a scorched-earth policy to protect his city.

∿, 📖, 🌀, ☺(∿ ✦)

= King, Talk, Burn, Calm (King City)

= The king ordered burning to calm his city

= The king ordered a scorched earth policy to protect his city

This answer is only a loose translation, but is the only option of those listed that comes close to translating the code.

15. A: Ride to the king as fast as you can!

● ✗↗☞, ∿

= You Ride Quickly, King

= Ride to the king as fast as you can!

Scorched earth

The term 'scorched-earth policy' originates from the policy of a retreating army burning all the crops to deprive an invading army of that food source. The policy was ruthless, because it guaranteed widespread starvation in one's own land, even if the invader was subsequently repelled. Nowadays, the term is a metaphor to describe an equally ruthless policy designed to spite others at considerable personal cost.

16. E: ✞ ❖ , ◌ ♌

Burn the Vatican City immediately! = Pope Home, Burn Now

= Burn the Pope's home now

= Burn the Vatican City immediately!

17. C: We're trapped; it's now every man for himself.

(◉ ●)(♉ ♇), ♌(◉ , ● , ■)

= (I You) (Run Negative), Now (I, You, He)

= We (cannot run), it's now all of us separate

= We're trapped; it's now every man for himself

18. D: You're all cowards; I'll fight again another day.

♇(● ●), ◉ ⧗(☹ 🔪 ☀)

= Cowardly (You You), I Then (Angry Kill)

= You all are cowardly; I will later fight

= You're all cowards; I'll fight again another day

19. B: If we bankrupt the king, we may still win.

♎(⌔ ⧗ ❄), (◉ ●) ➑ ♪

= Conditional (King Then Poor), (I You) Take Positive

= If the king is then poor, we will be able to take successfully

= If we bankrupt the king, we may still win

20. E: The peasants are taxed excessively by both church and state.

    ◆◆, ✉✍✍, ᎣↃ✝

    = Peasant Peasant, Pay Positive Positive, King Pope

    = Peasants, pay a lot, state church

    = The peasants are taxed excessively by both church and state

21. A: The queen paid the cardinal to keep her affair with the king's chief knight a secret.

    ♍, ✉, 📖, ♎, ☝📖, ♍(ᎣↃ(☞✍))

    = Queen, Pay, Cardinal, Negative Talk, Queen (King (Knight Positive))

    = The queen paid the cardinal to not talk about queen (king's chief knight)

    = The queen paid the cardinal to not talk about the queen with king's chief knight

    = The queen paid the cardinal to keep her affair with the king's chief knight a secret

22. B: Internet

    And

    C: Television

    You can encode the word 'politician' with 'talk knight' or 'talk peasant', depending on your level of respect for politicians. The term 'road tours' may be 'ride quickly' – or even 'ride quickly, peasant peasant home' if you want to convey a sense of visiting the electorate. Finally, you can substitute 'talk' for 'communicate'.

    Conveying the word 'internet' or 'television' effectively without new code is much harder.

23. D: ❽, ♌⧗(✍, ☞, ✿✍, ❄✍, ◗☄➹, ☺✍)

    = Take, Now Then (Positive, Negative, Rich Positive, Poor Positive, Kill Slowly, Calm Positive)

    = Have by taking, from this day forward (good, bad, richer, poorer, ill, well)

    = To have and to hold, from this day forward, for better, for worse, for richer, for poorer, in sickness, and in health

    This phrase is an excerpt from the traditional marriage vows.

24. C: ☺(☺◌), ⌛(♎, ♎◌)

   = Calm (Calm Positive), Then (Conditional, Conditional Negative)

   = Calm (Happy), Then (may be, may be not)

   = Let be happy, future may be or may not be

   = Whoever wants to be happy, let him be so: of tomorrow there's no knowing

   This phrase is a partial quote from Lorenzo de' Medici, also known as Lorenzo the Magnificent, de facto ruler of Renaissance Florence. His death marked the end of the Golden Age of Florence, making the quote even more poignant.

25. B: ⌂❖, ◌❖(✧✧)

   = Cardinal Home, Cowardly Home (Rich Rich)

   = Cardinal's home is cowardly home of riches

   = The cardinal's palace is the cowardly home of gold

   = The gold is hidden in the cardinal's palace

26. C: ♞, ↗☞. ◌(✝⌂⌂), ☯

   = Knight, Ride Quickly, Negative (Pope Cardinal Cardinal), Burn

   = The knight charged on horseback, Negative (god's church), Burn

   = The knight charged on horseback, satanic cult, burning

   = The knight charged on horseback into the satanic cult's fire

27. B: If the Pope dies, the cardinal will become Pope.

   ♎,✝,💣※,⌂,♎,✝

   = Conditional, Pope Kill, Cardinal, Conditional, Pope

   = If the Pope dies, the cardinal will become Pope.

   This sentence is the only one that uses the conditional twice and 'pope' twice, as per the code.

28. D: The cardinal sailed to Rome for an audience with the Pope.

   ⌂,〰,✝,📖,✝

   = Cardinal, Sail, Pope, Talk, Pope

   The first 'Pope' is used as a synonym for Rome. 'Talk' conveys the desire for an audience.

   = The cardinal sailed to Rome for an audience with the Pope.

Situational Judgement Test

1, A; **2**, A; **3**, D; **4**, D

Discussion:

By exploring Mrs Jones's concerns about receiving home help, Mr Jones may be able to allay her fears or reservations and negotiate a solution (item 1). By having a conversation with her, he can also explore acceptable alternatives to home help, such as staying with a friend or relative (item 2).

To delay Mrs Jones's discharge on non-medical grounds (item 3) would be very inappropriate, because it would be an ineffective use of a bed, and, by extension, of public money.

To immediately discharge Mrs Jones on the assumption that she has mental capacity (item 4) is irresponsible, particularly since Mr Digby hasn't taken the trouble to formally assess her mental capacity. Even if Mrs Jones does have full mental capacity, Mr Digby ought to try to negotiate some sort of acceptable solution.

5, C; **6**, A; **7**, D; **8**, A; **9**, D

Discussion:

To ask the neighbours about John's whereabouts (item 5) would be inappropriate, since it would let them know, or at least suspect, that John's mentally ill and in need of psychiatric assessment.

To try to ascertain John's whereabouts by calling his nearest relative (most likely his mother or father) or John himself (items 6 and 8) is very appropriate and may help to quickly resolve the situation.

To force entry to the property (item 7) would be a gross overreaction at this stage, and it would also require a court order.

To aim to return in one month's time (item 9) would be very inappropriate, because John may be mentally ill and at risk to himself and others. Ideally, the mental health team should aim to return later that same day.

10, D; **11**, A; **12**, A

Discussion:

John clearly represents a real degree of risk to the mental health team. To insist on assessing him in these circumstances (item 10) would put the mental health team in potential danger. Instead, the team should leave without delay and return later with more people and security (items 11 and 12).

13, A; **14**, A; **15**, A; **16**, C

Discussion:

Mrs Bridgens is likely to be suffering from depression, in which case she may commit suicide regardless of the likely outcome (or prognosis) of the breast cancer. For this reason, the patient's likelihood of recovering from breast cancer (item 16) isn't an important factor in determining her current risk of suicide.

On the other hand, Mrs Bridgens' risk of committing suicide is strongly influenced by her degree of intent (how strongly she wants to do it), her mental state (for example, whether or not she is suffering from depression), and her level of social support (whether somebody is able to watch her and make sure that she's safe) (questions 13, 14 and 15). If Mrs Bridgens presents an overall high risk of suicide, the GP ought to refer her for a psychiatric assessment with a view to possible hospital admission.

17, A; **18**, A; **19**, A; **20**, D

Discussion:

People with a psychotic illness should stop driving during a first psychotic episode or psychotic relapse of their illness, because driving can seriously endanger lives. In the UK, such people must notify the Driver and Vehicle Licensing Agency (DVLA).

Broadly speaking, the psychiatrist can reinstate a patient's licence if satisfied that the patient no longer presents a danger to himself or herself or to other road users.

Central to the psychiatrist's decision to reinstate Lucy's driving licence is her current mental state (whether she's currently well), her compliance with her medication (since good compliance minimises the chances of another imminent relapse), and the nature and degree of any medication side effects that she may be suffering from (since side effects such as dizziness or sedation are likely to increase her risk) (items 17, 18 and 19).

The psychiatrist should not factor in to the decision the extent to which Lucy needs to drive (item 20), which ought to be made on the grounds of safety alone.

21, A; **22**, D; **23**, D; **24**, A

Discussion:

Adults are entitled to refuse potentially life-saving treatment, although a special consent form is required. Doctors must be satisfied that patients are aware of the risks involved in refusing treatment, and that there's no coercion (item 21). Because Dr Banerjee is a junior doctor, he ought to seek advice from a senior colleague (item 24) and possibly also from his defence body.

To challenge a person's religious views (item 23), however unreasonable they may seem, is certainly not the place of a medical professional. To discharge Linda at this point (item 22) would be very dangerous, as she could potentially collapse in the street.

25, D; **26**, A; **27**, A

Discussion:

It's a criminal offence to ill-treat, neglect or abandon a child under the age of 16. If James were to die, Dr Banerjee could be liable to a charge of manslaughter. Witholding treatment is therefore very inappropriate, making D the answer to Item 25.

In the past, James would have been made a ward of court. Nowadays, the clinician, preferably a consultant, simply instigates treatment on the grounds that this is in the child's best interests. Sometimes, treatment is delivered under a so-called Specific Issue Order. Answers 26 and 27 highlight the appropriateness of urgently seeking good advice.

28, B; **29**, C; **30**, A; **31**, D

Discussion:

The first thing to realise is that Arun will take not more than two minutes to help this patient who, with his Zimmer frame and cardiac complaint, can't afford to get lost.

The second thing to realise is that Arun's in the hospital in his capacity as a medical student, and must try to behave as a future doctor might. Ideally, he should give the patient careful directions and then excuse himself to his supervisor for being late, perhaps even explaining why he's late (item 30).

To politely apologise to the patient and explain that he's in a hurry (item 28) is fine, but is a little lacking in perspective. To do no more than wave at the overhead signs (item 29) is a bit dismissive of the patient, who, in addition, may not be able to see, read, or understand the signs. To ignore the patient (item 31) is simply rude and reflects very poorly on a future doctor.

32, A; **33**, B; **34**, C; **35**, C; **36**, D

Discussion:

In this situation, it's best to act immediately and, if possible, discretely, to protect the confidentiality of the patients being discussed (item 32). It's also important to remind the medical students in question that their behaviour, though more careless than malign, is unacceptable. This should prevent such a situation from arising in the future.

To wait until the medical students are out of the lift and then have a word with them (item 33) *does* address their behaviour, but not quite soon enough.

Obviously, to do nothing (item 36) achieves none of this.

To subtly change the subject of the conversation (item 34) is nothing but a stopgap measure that fails to address the behaviour of the medical students. To report them to the senior tutor (item 35) at this early stage would be an overreaction.

37, A; **38**, A; **39**, A; **40**, A

Discussion:

Doctors should treat their patients with respect, whatever the patients' lifestyle choices and beliefs (item 37). All patients are entitled to care and treatment, regardless of whether they are deemed responsible for their plight (item 38).

Ideally, doctors should be able to practise in accordance with their beliefs (item 39), provided that patients receive effective and timely care and aren't discriminated against. General Medical Council (GMC) guidance allows doctors the right to say no to a particular procedure, but not to a particular patient or group of patients. In this case, Dr Cosgrove can explain her personal beliefs to Clarissa, as long as she's careful not to cause Clarissa any further distress (item 40). Dr Cosgrove can also refer Clarissa to another GP, although, in this case, GMC guidance doesn't require it.

In an emergency, the GMC expects doctors to set aside their personal beliefs to provide effective patient care.

41, A; **42**, B; **43**, D; **44**, A

Discussion:

Doctors must provide or arrange treatment for a patient only if it's to the overall physical or psychological benefit of the patient (item 41). While a patient's request for treatment (item 42) does have some part to play, it shouldn't override the doctor's professional judgement.

Whether the patient is paying for the procedure (item 43) is irrelevant, because this isn't a matter of cost but of ethics.

While patients are entitled to approach specialists directly and to withhold this from their GP, specialists need access to the patient's historical information (item 44) so as to assess the risk of the procedure.

45, A; **46**, B; **47**, D; **48**, B

Discussion:

Doctors must always act in the best interests of children and young people (item 45), even if, as in this case, the child's best interests are difficult to determine. While Will, at 6 years old, probably doesn't have the capacity to decide for himself, his views are important and should be taken into account (item 46).

Divorce or separation doesn't affect parental responsibility, and everyone with parental responsibility should be involved in any important discussions about their child's treatment (item 47). In this case, Dr Alcock ought to work with the parents to reach some sort of consensus.

Seeking the views of a third party (item 48) will help to achieve a consensus as well as give a clearer picture of where Will's best interests lie. If a consensus can't be achieved, it may be necessary to go down the legal route.

49, A; **50**, A; **51**, D; **52**, A; **53**, D

Discussion:

It's important to be open and honest with patients if things go wrong. If a patient under a doctor's care has suffered harm or distress, the doctor must offer an apology (item 49), explain fully and promptly what's happened (item 50), and try in as far as possible to put matters right (item 52).

A doctor should only end a professional relationship with a patient (item 51) when the breakdown of trust between the doctor and the patient means that the doctor can no longer provide good clinical care to the patient.

In this case, to suggest that Mrs Chalmers' behaviour is unreasonable (item 53) is inappropriate; that's for somebody else or other people to decide.

54, C; **55**, A; **56**, A; **57**, C; **58**, C

Discussion:

The type of work that Mr Fulford undertakes – and, ultimately, the safety of his patients – are paramount in this case (items 55 and 56). The severity of Mr Fulford's condition (item 54) is of only minor importance, because it's already been established that he occasionally suffers from sleep attacks, and a single sleep attack could spell the death of one of his patients.

Mr Fulford's response to treatment (item 57) is important, but this can only be fully assessed over a relatively long period. Meanwhile, Mr Fulford is at least theoretically vulnerable to further sleep attacks.

Finally, it would be polite and considerate to ask Mr Fulford for his opinion (item 58), but, ultimately, Dr Vasanti needs to act on the facts alone.

Mr Fulford's employer needs to be made aware of his condition so that appropriate measures can be taken to ensure the safety of Mr Fulford's patients.

59, D; **60**, C; **61**, A; **62**, A; **63**, A

Discussion:

A health professional who thinks that patient safety, dignity or comfort is seriously compromised must take prompt action (item 59). If a patient's not receiving basic care, the health professional must immediately tell someone who's in a position to act immediately (item 62).

Because Dr Chan's a junior doctor and new to the ward, it's a good idea for him to first discuss the issue with his consultant (item 61).

To carry out an audit of basic care on the ward (item 63) is an excellent way both to assess the scale of the problem and to make the nursing staff more aware and more engaged. This need not preclude dealing with the situation immediately.

Finally, Dr Chan ought to try to resolve matters internally before calling the Care Quality Commission (item 60).

64, A; **65**, A; **66**, A; **67**, A; **68**, C

Discussion:

It's very important to have a frank discussion with Foster's parents, who may have legitimate concerns about divulging the diagnosis (item 64). The parents' wishes ought to be taken into account, but Dr Shah's primary duty is to her patient, Foster (item 68).

Conversely, it's very important to assess Foster's capacity, and, indeed, his desire to understand his diagnosis and its implications; if Foster doesn't have the capacity or the desire to know his diagnosis, Dr Shah will do him more harm than good by revealing it to him (items 65 and 66).

Whether to divulge or hold back a diagnosis from a young child is a thorny issue, particularly if the child's parents are asking for it to be withheld. In such circumstances, Dr Shah would be well advised to consult the GMC's guidelines (item 67).

69, A; **70**, A; **71**, C

Discussion:

Nathan's right to confidentiality is paramount and must be maintained unless someone else is at risk (item 69). Someone is certainly at risk if Nathan has had or intends to have unprotected sexual intercourse with either of his partners (item 70).

It's not for Dr Sharma to pass open judgement on Nathan's lifestyle. The fact that he has two partners is important only in that it suggests that Nathan's promiscuous and so more likely to be putting others at risk of infection (item 71). There's also the further question of how Nathan contracted HIV/AIDS. Either he contracted it from one of his partners, in which case his partners also need to be tested, or he contracted it from outside those relationships. It may be possible to test Nathan's partners while still preserving Nathan's confidentiality.

Chapter 11

Practice Test Two

In This Chapter

▶ Doing a complete timed UKCAT practice test

This test is the second of two complete UKCAT practice tests that we include in this book (the other complete test is in Chapter 9). You can do the two tests in any order. They both stand up on their own as a way of doing lots of practice questions under timed conditions.

We recommend that you work through this test in one session, allocating the right amount of time to each part of the test. (We show the UKCAT subtest timings in the table below.)

Timings for the UKCAT Subtests	
Subtest	**Time Allowed**
Verbal reasoning	22 minutes
Quantitative reasoning	23 minutes
Abstract reasoning	14 minutes
Decision analysis	34 minutes
Situational judgement test	27 minutes

If you have special educational needs and plan to sit the UKCATSEN, you can give yourself an extra 25 per cent of time. (For more about the UKCATSEN, see Chapter 2.)

In Chapter 12, we give the answers and full explanations for the questions in this practice test.

Verbal Reasoning

High Noon

(Adapted from *Celestial Navigation* by Tom Cunliffe)

Local noon occurs at the moment when the Sun, on its journey from east to west, crosses the observer's meridian. At any one time, you are on a particular terrestrial meridian of longitude. When the Sun bears exactly due south or due north of you, or once in a lifetime is right over your head (at your zenith), its celestial meridian (its Greenwich Hour Angle) will correspond to your longitude.

As we are about to see, if you can observe the altitude of any celestial body when it is exactly on your meridian, a surprisingly simple calculation leads to the latitude. Since finding this is half the battle, and because the Sun is very much in evidence at noon, the noon sight has always been the cornerstone of the navigator's day.

Obviously, the Greenwich time of noon is going to vary from location to location as the Sun appears to travel around the Earth. When you are sitting on deck with your sextant, you can tell when the Sun has reached its noon altitude because it doesn't get any higher. Nevertheless, you don't want to be hanging around all day waiting for it, so it helps to work out the approximate time of local noon.

1. The celestial meridian at noon corresponds to your longitude.

   A. True
   B. False
   C. Can't tell

2. The noon sighting of the Sun is important to navigators because it allows them to calculate their position.

   A. True
   B. False
   C. Can't tell

3. The Sun is at your zenith when it's directly beneath you.

   A. True
   B. False
   C. Can't tell

4. The Earth revolves around the Sun.

   A. True
   B. False
   C. Can't tell

This Isn't Just Food . . .

**(Adapted from *Never Mind the Sizzle . . . Where's the Sausage?*
by David J Taylor)**

I got some welcome inspiration from a Marks & Spencer's chocolate pudding advert Claire and I saw on Saturday night. In contrast to our pizza ad, the second this one started I knew which brand it was for. I recognised the music, although it was almost drowned out by the moans and groans that Claire was making next to me on the sofa. Her reaction was understandable, as the chocolate pudding in question did look amazing. The film did a great job of celebrating the product, taking time to show a fork appearing and then piercing the pud with a river of steaming sauce pouring out. The languorous voice-over then told us that 'This isn't just food; this is M&S food.' It was more than that even; it was food porn.

The effectiveness of the commercial was confirmed in two ways. First, when we sat down to dinner after the kids had finally gone to bed, we had M&S chocolate pud for dessert. Second, and more importantly, a quick bit of Googling led me to the news that M&S and their agency had won the Grand Prix for their work, which had played a major role in the brand's turnaround and increased pudding sales by a whopping 288%!

5. Brand awareness can be reinforced by an easily recognisable soundtrack.

   A. True
   B. False
   C. Can't tell

6. An advertising campaign needs to target women like Claire.

   A. True
   B. False
   C. Can't tell

7. Marks & Spencer's advertising campaign led to a 288 per cent increase in food sales.

   A. True
   B. False
   C. Can't tell

8. The author is impressed by M&S's advertising.

   A. True
   B. False
   C. Can't tell

Independence

(Adapted from *The Unauthorized Guide to Doing Business the Simon Cowell Way* by Trevor Clawson)

As he continues to grow his global television and music interests, Simon Cowell is in an enviable position. He's rich. He has a close and mutually beneficial commercial relationship with Sony. And, above all, he's in control of his own destiny to a degree that most people in and outside of the music and entertainment industries can only dream of.

But Cowell's autonomy has been hard won. His early attempts to work independently of the big guns of the record industry ended in failure. Since then Cowell has adopted a different strategy. Rather than working independently of the music industry, he built his businesses in partnership with a corporate. First with BMG and now with Sony, while remaining a high-profile leader rather than a cog in the bigger machine. It's a neat trick.

His 50–50 joint venture with Sony, Syco, is an example of enlightened self-interest in action. From Sony's perspective, Cowell is one of a rare breed of golden geese laying golden eggs. Meanwhile, Cowell continues to work with a company that has the resources to help him put his ideas into practice, and his name remains firmly above the door of Syco for the foreseeable future.

The upshot of all this is that Cowell is a living embodiment of the old maxim: You don't get rich on a salary.

9. Simon Cowell has more autonomy than most music professionals.

   A. True
   B. False
   C. Can't tell

10. Simon Cowell is profitable for Sony.

   A. True
   B. False
   C. Can't tell

11. Simon Cowell has always been successful.

   A. True
   B. False
   C. Can't tell

12. According to the author, self-interest underpins Simon Cowell's relatively large degree of personal autonomy in his relationship with Sony.

   A. True
   B. False
   C. Can't tell

You Will Be Assimilated!

(Adapted from *Sociology For Dummies* by Nasar Meer and Jay Gabler)

Not all ethnic groups are immigrant groups – most societies have a number of indigenous ethnic groups as well as ethnic groups that have come from elsewhere, plus there are ethnic groups not associated with a place of origin. Still, almost all sociologists interested in race and ethnicity find themselves looking closely at the experiences of immigrants.

The members of the Chicago School were among the first sociologists to really look closely at immigration. The turn of the 20th century saw a wave of immigration to the United States that transformed America's social landscape, and that transformation was most visible in big cities like Chicago, where the new arrivals went looking for work.

Initially, sociologists thought immigration could be understood in terms of 'assimilation'. The word assimilation means to be absorbed into, to become one of. America was seen as a great 'melting pot' where people from all different places arrived to be incorporated into one big whole.

The theory of assimilation has it that people arrive speaking their native languages, wearing their native styles of dress, and otherwise practising the traditions of their home countries. Over time, they are assimilated into their new community, adopting that country's language and traditions. If that's the way it works, the study of immigration is just the study of why some groups assimilate more quickly and peacefully than others.

13. Immigration can result in the arrival of new ethnic groups into a society.

   A. True
   B. False
   C. Can't tell

14. Immigration is largely driven by economic factors.

   A. True
   B. False
   C. Can't tell

15. Assimilation assumes that the eventual outcome of immigration is integration into the existing community's traditions.

   A. True
   B. False
   C. Can't tell

16. The study of immigration is the study of why some groups assimilate more quickly and peacefully than others.

   A. True
   B. False
   C. Can't tell

Get Me the Best You Have

(Adapted from *The Unauthorized Guide To Doing Business the Jamie Oliver Way* by Trevor Clawson)

Oliver has not been slow to recruit big hitters into all parts of his organisation and to work with strong personalities.

As the commissioning editor at Channel 4 and series producer on *Jamie's School Dinners* says, Oliver knows when to delegate to other people: 'The thing about Jamie is he spots talent, recognises what everyone else's strengths are and then lets you do what you're good at. He understood we needed great TV moments, as programme makers.'

Away from the camera, Oliver has appointed expert managers to his businesses. They have included David Page, formerly managing director of Indian food company Patak, who joined Oliver's Fresh Retail Ventures in 2007. He wasted no time in signalling his plans to take the company on a fast growth curve.

Oliver's TV production company also has an experienced hand at the helm. Recruited from Diverse Productions – a key supplier of programmes to Channel 4 – Roy Ackerman joined Fresh One with a brief to diversify from a portfolio of shows that were largely centred around Oliver.

Employing high flyers as managers is about more than putting the day-to-day management of a growing business in safe hands. They bring in expertise in their chosen industries, coupled with their own managerial skills. They also make a business more sustainable and in some cases saleable.

17. Channel 4's commissioning editor believes that great TV moments are essential to programme making.

    A. True
    B. False
    C. Can't tell

18. Roy Ackerman plans to make more shows centred around Jamie Oliver.

    A. True
    B. False
    C. Can't tell

19. High-flying managers have the potential to increase an owner's wealth.

    A. True
    B. False
    C. Can't tell

20. Fresh Retail Ventures has been on a fast growth curve since 2007.

    A. True
    B. False
    C. Can't tell

Digital Pennies

(Adapted from *Socialnomics* by Erik Qualman)

It's inevitable that all of our broadcasts will eventually be pushed through the internet and a majority will be viewed on tablets and iPads. Brand budgets that historically went to television, magazine ads, and outdoor boards are moving to digital channels for three main reasons: 1) the audience has moved there, 2) it's more cost-effective, and 3) it's easier to track. What will happen?

In the short-term there will be companies that are able to take advantage of this transition. Just as online travel agents were able to take advantage for suppliers and make a slow progression to web bookings, aggressive conduit companies will be able to deliver what the audience wants. The same holds true for online distributors of music jumping on the opportunity made available by the ineptness of the music industry to embrace digital music.

At the beginning of 2008, Jeff Zucker, the boss of NBC Universal, told an audience of TV executives that their biggest challenge was to ensure 'that we do not end up trading analogue dollars for digital pennies.' Zucker understood that the audience was moving online faster than advertisers were, thus leaving media companies in a position of possibly losing advertising revenue and having their inventory devalued if and when they moved online with their TV content.

21. It's inevitable that most broadcasts will be watched on iPads.

   A. True
   B. False
   C. Can't tell

22. The ability to track digital channels is a key reason behind a shift in advertising budgets to the digital sphere.

   A. True
   B. False
   C. Can't tell

23. Viewer numbers and advertising budgets do not necessarily move synchronously to fresh platforms.

   A. True
   B. False
   C. Can't tell

24. Eventually, online broadcasters should be able to attract roughly comparable revenue to normal TV broadcasters.

   A. True
   B. False
   C. Can't tell

Taking Advantage

(Adapted from *The Art of War* by Sun Tzu)

If the enemy be at rest in comfortable quarters, harass him; if he be living in plenty, cut off his supplies; if sitting composedly awaiting attack, cause him to move. This may be done by appearing where the enemy is not, and assaulting unexpected points.

If we go where the enemy is not, we may go a thousand leagues without exhaustion. If we attack those positions which the enemy has not defended, we invariably take them; but on defence we must be strong, even where we are not likely to be attacked.

Against those skilful in attack, the enemy does not know where to defend; against those skilful in defence, the enemy does not know where to attack.

Now the secrets of the art of offence are not to be easily apprehended, as a certain shape or noise can be understood, of the senses; but when these secrets are learnt, the enemy is mastered.

We attack, and the enemy cannot resist, because we attack his insufficiency; we retire and the enemy cannot pursue, because we retire too quickly.

The leader who changes his tactics in accordance with his adversary, and thereby controls the issue, may be called the God of War.

25. Sun Tzu recommends that you should defeat an opponent in an entrenched position by aggressively attacking him there.

   A. True
   B. False
   C. Can't tell

26. Mobility is an essential component of successful warfare.

   A. True
   B. False
   C. Can't tell

27. The lessons of *The Art of War* may be interpreted metaphorically for modern civilian life.

   A. True
   B. False
   C. Can't tell

28. To be successful in warfare requires a general to be flexible enough to respond to changing situations.

   A. True
   B. False
   C. Can't tell

Living Outside the Cave

(Adapted from *Plato: Letters to my Son* by Neel Burton)

Human beings are like prisoners in a cave, who have spent all their lives with their backs turned against its mouth. Their neck and legs have been chained up so that they cannot move and can only see in front of them, that is, towards the back of the cave. Above and behind them is a blazing fire, and between them and the fire is a ramp with a low wall. Little men, who are hidden behind the low wall, scuttle along the ramp carrying all sorts of statues upon their heads, and the fire casts the shadows of the statues onto the back of the cave. As the prisoners only ever see the shadows, they naturally come to believe that the shadows are the objects themselves. When a prisoner is unshackled and turned towards the fire, he suffers sharp pains, but after some time his eyes accommodate to the light and, for the first time, he is then dragged out of the cave, where objects are real and not mere statues or replicas. But here the light is so bright that he cannot gaze upon any actual objects, and must train his eyes, first upon shadows and then upon reflections. In time, he finally looks up into the sky and understands that the sun is the cause of everything that he sees around him, of light, of vision, and of the objects of vision. The purpose of education is to drag the prisoner as far out of the cave as possible, not to show him this or that particular object, but to turn his whole soul towards the sun.

29. Which of the following does not describe the conditions in the cave?

A. The prisoners are accustomed to darkness.

B. The back of the cave is like a screen onto which the shadows of statues are reflected.

C. The prisoners are unaware of what is going on behind them.

D. A blazing fire is in front of a ramp with a low wall.

30. Which of the following can be inferred from the passage?

A. The prisoners are reluctant to leave the cave.

B. The prisoners are keen to leave the cave.

C. Some prisoners who leave the cave go blind.

D. When a prisoner who escaped from the cave returns to tell the other prisoners what he's seen, he's treated like a madman.

31. Which statement is the author least likely to agree with?

A. The shadows on the back of the cave are shadows of replicas and not of real objects.

B. A prisoner who manages to leave the cave is unlikely to want to return.

C. Education is a matter of learning facts.

D. Education is a matter of seeing more clearly.

32. The passage is best described as:

A. A story

B. A myth

C. A fable

D. An allegory

Indestructible

(Adapted from *Wine For Dummies* by Ed McCarthy and Mary Ewing-Mulligan)

The legendary wine called Madeira comes from the island of the same name, which sits in the Atlantic Ocean nearer to Africa than Europe. Madeira is a subtropical island whose precarious hillside vineyards rise straight up from the ocean. The island is a province of Portugal, but the British have always run its wine trade. Historically, Madeira could even be considered something of an American wine, for this is the wine that American Colonists drank.

Madeira can lay claim to being the world's longest-lived wine. A few years ago, we were fortunate enough to try a 1799 Vintage Madeira that was still perfectly fine. Only Hungary's Tokaji Azsu can rival Madeira in longevity, and that's true only of its rarest examples, such as its Essencia.

Although Madeira's fortified wines were quite the rage 200 years ago, the island's vineyards were devastated at the end of the 19th century, first by mildew and then by the phylloxera louse. Most vineyards were replanted with lesser grapes. The very best Madeira wines are still those from the old days, vintage-dated wines from 1920 back to 1795. The prices aren't outrageous either (£200–£300 a bottle), considering what other wines that old, such as Bordeaux, cost.

33. Madeira is a British–American wine.

    A. True

    B. False

    C. Can't tell

34. Madeira lasts centuries because it's already undergone oxidisation.

    A. True

    B. False

    C. Can't tell

35. Phylloxera devastated the wine industry towards the end of the 19th century.

    A. True

    B. False

    C. Can't tell

36. A vintage Madeira is good value for money compared with Bordeaux.

    A. True

    B. False

    C. Can't tell

Capitalist Communists

(Adapted from *An Introduction to the Chinese Economy* by Rongxing Guo)

While China's reform has been a strong driver of its economic growth, it has also derived a series of socioeconomic problems. Prior to the reform, China was an egalitarian society in terms of income distribution. In the initial stage of the reform, the policy of 'letting some people get rich first' *(rang yi bufen ren xian fui qilai)* was adopted in order to overcome egalitarianism in income distribution, to promote efficiency with strong incentives, and ultimately realise common prosperity based on an enlarged pie. But this policy has quickly enlarged income gaps between different groups of people.

According to the Gini coefficient, China has very high levels of inequality, only lower than a few nations in Latin America and Africa. However, there is a different view with respect to this issue: that China's current income inequality has been overestimated and, if measured in terms of purchasing power parity (PPP) rates, China's apparent income inequality should be reduced considerably, as in most cases the price levels in poor areas are much lower than those in rich areas.

37. China has moved at least some of the way towards a capitalist economic structure.

   A. True
   B. False
   C. Can't tell

38. Income inequality is an inevitable function of a liberalising economy.

   A. True
   B. False
   C. Can't tell

39. PPP is a better measure of income inequality than is the Gini coefficient.

   A. True
   B. False
   C. Can't tell

40. If inflation increases in China, it negatively impacts the poorest in China.

   A. True
   B. False
   C. Can't tell

All Good Things

(Adapted from *Aristotle's Universe* by Neel Burton)

Near the end of his life, Alexander the Great ordered the execution as a traitor of Aristotle's grandnephew Callisthenes and this and other things soured the relationship between the king and his master.

After Alexander's death in Babylon in 323 BC, anti-Macedonian feelings in Athens flared up, and Eurydemon the hierophant denounced Aristotle for not holding the gods in honour. Aristotle fled to his country house at Chalcis on Euboea, an island off the Attic coast and the homeland of his mother's family. Referring to the trial and execution of Socrates in 399 BC, he famously explained, 'I will not allow the Athenians to sin twice against philosophy'.

He died of an abdominal complaint within the year on March 7 of 322 BC, aged sixty-two. There is a story according to which he threw himself into the sea 'because he could not explain the tides', but this is unlikely to be true, as are other fanciful conjectures about his death.

After Aristotle left Athens, Theophrastus – who was not Macedonian but Lesbian – became *scholarch* (leader) of the peripatetic school, and in his will Aristotle made provisions for him and for others to take over the care of his children and of Herpyllis. He also left him his works and his library, and designated him as head of the Lyceum.

41. In the first sentence, 'his master' most likely refers to:

    A. Aristotle

    B. Alexander

    C. Callisthenes

    D. Socrates

42. From the information in the passage, which of the following is true?

    A. Alexander and Aristotle never got on well.

    B. Alexander died from natural causes.

    C. Aristotle thought he'd be safe on Euboea.

    D. Aristotle had met with Socrates.

43. Which of the following can be inferred from the passage?

    A. The Lyceum is another name for the peripatetic school.

    B. Alexander disliked Aristotle.

    C. Aristotle was born on Euboea.

    D. After Alexander's death, Aristotle feared for his life.

44. From the information in the passage, which of the following is least likely?

    A. Aristotle disliked Theophrastus.

    B. Eurydemon the hierophant disliked Macedonians.

    C. Most people living in those times were fairly religious.

    D. Aristotle was a philosopher.

Quantitative Reasoning

MPs' Expenses

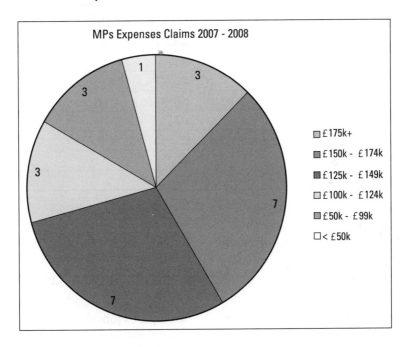

MPs Expenses Claims 2007 - 2008

■ £175k+
■ £150k - £174k
■ £125k - £149k
□ £100k - £124k
■ £50k - £99k
□ < £50k

MPs' expense claims were leaked to the press. The figure shows the amounts claimed by a representative sample of 24 MPs (k = £1,000).

1. Approximately what percentage of MPs claimed at least £125k?

(A) 12.5%   (B) 29.2%
(C) 41.7%   (D) 70.8%   (E) 82.3%

2. What's the ratio of MPs claiming £150k or more to those claiming less than £150k?

(A) 1:7   (B) 5:7   (C) 17:7
(D) 5:12   (E) 1:8

3. The MPs in the £100k–£124k category claimed a total of £340k between them. If the MP with the largest claim in this category claimed £121k, what's the maximum that one of the other MPs in this category may have claimed?

(A) £100k   (B) £105.5k
(C) £109.5k   (D) £119k   (E) £124k

4. MPs have reduced their expense claims by 19 per cent since a new system for making claims was introduced. If the previous total bill for all 650 MPs was £98 million per year, what's the new annual total? Round your answer to the nearest million pounds.

(A) £19 million   (B) £28 million
(C) £62 million   (D) £79 million
(E) £81 million

US Jobs Data

The table shows US Monthly Employment Gains.

US Monthly Employment Gains	
Month	**Jobs Added (Thousands)**
January	68
February	235
March	194
April	217
May	53
June	46
July	117

5. What's the average number of jobs added per month, in thousands, to the nearest thousand?

(A) 78   (B) 93   (C) 115
(D) 133   (E) 235

6. In what month was the 600,000th new job added in the year?

(A) February   (B) March
(C) April   (D) May   (E) June

7. What was the approximate ratio of new jobs added in June and July versus those added in January and February?

(A) 1:1   (B) 1:1.9   (C) 1:2.2
(D) 1:3   (E) 1:7

8. August's jobs data shows a 23 per cent increase over the average of the second quarter of the year. Approximately how many jobs were added in August, in thousands?

(A) 89   (B) 105   (C) 130
(D) 144   (E) 204

Inflation in the East

The table shows inflation rates in Asian economies.

Inflation Rates in Asian Economies (%)							
Japan	0.2	Singapore	5.2	Malaysia	3.1	Bangladesh	10.2
Philippines	4.0	India	8.6	Kazakhstan	8.5	Thailand	4.1
Sri Lanka	7.5	Taiwan	1.3	Hong Kong	5.6	China	6.5
Vietnam	22.2	South Korea	4.7	Pakistan	13.8	Indonesia	4.6

A first-year analyst at an investment bank is asked to categorise the data into bands based on the inflation rate. He draws up the following table.

Asian Inflation, by Band	
Band	*Number of Countries*
0–4.9%	7
5.0–9.9%	6
10.0–14.9%	2
>15%	2

9. Is there anything wrong with Table 11-4?

A. One too few in the 0–4.9% band
B. One too many in the 0–4.9% band
C. One too many in the >15% band
D. One too few in the >15% band
E. No – nothing's wrong with the table

10. What's the approximate average inflation rate of those countries in the 5.0–9.9 per cent band?

(A) 5.4% (B) 6% (C) 7%
(D) 7.3% (E) 7.5%

11. By what percentage does Japan's inflation rate have to increase to match South Korea's?

(A) 2% (B) 4.5% (C) 91%
(D) 2,150% (E) 2,250%

12. India's GDP is $1.4 trillion. China's GDP is $5 trillion. What's the average rate of inflation across these two countries, assuming that the impact of each country's rate of inflation on the combined countries' rate of inflation is proportional to the GDP of that country's economy?

(A) 7% (B) 7.2 % (C) 7.4%
(D) 7.6% (E) 25.6%

0. 043

Under Par

The table is a sample of the total number of strokes taken by 20 players at the US PGA golf major tournament.

US PGA Total Scores				
276	283	290	273	285
285	290	272	286	295
291	272	294	284	275
281	285	288	277	280

13. What score is the modal average?

(A) 272   (B) 276   (C) 280
(D) 285   (E) 290

14. What's the mean score? Round your answer to the nearest whole stroke.

(A) 277   (B) 279   (C) 281
(D) 282   (E) 283

15. What percentage of scores are less than 286?

(A) 55%   (B) 60%   (C) 65%
(D) 70%   (E) 75%

16. The top two players, KB and JD, are tied at 272 strokes, and go on to a play-off over a further three holes. The odds of player KB winning the play-off are 5:11. Express these odds as a percentage chance of winning, rounding your answer to the nearest whole percentage.

(A) 19%   (B) 31%   (C) 45%
(D) 69%   (E) 81%

The Winner's Circle

Questions 17–20 refer to horse racing.

Horse races use imperial units of measurement: 1 mile = 8 furlongs = 1,760 yards.

17. The Epsom Derby is held over 12 furlongs. In 2011, Pour Moi completed the course to win in 2 minutes and 35 seconds. How fast is Pour Moi's speed in miles per hour (mph)? Round your answer to the nearest whole number.

    (A) 15   (B) 23   (C) 35
    (D) 184   (E) 279

18. The third-placed horse, the Queen's Carlton House, finished 5 yards back from the winner mentioned in item 17. In what time did it complete the course, assuming that Carlton House maintained a steady speed throughout the race? Round your answer to the first decimal place.

    A. 155.1 seconds
    B. 155.3 seconds
    C. 155.5 seconds
    D. 156.1 seconds
    E. 156.7 seconds

19. The fastest ever Derby-winning time was 2 minutes and 31 seconds, recorded by Workforce in 2010. Assuming uniform speeds, by what approximate distance did Workforce beat Pour Moi?

    (A) 62 yards   (B) 64 yards
    (C) 66 yards   (D) 68 yards
    (E) 70 yards

20. The St Leger Stakes are held later in the year than the Derby, on a course measuring 1 mile, 6 furlongs and 132 yards. If a horse wins the St Leger by travelling at the same average speed as Pour Moi did when winning the Derby, what's its approximate winning time?

    A. 2 minutes 50 seconds
    B. 2 minutes 51 seconds
    C. 2 minutes 55 seconds
    D. 3 minutes
    E. 3 minutes 9 seconds

Eating into the Market

The figure below shows the changing market shares of three major UK supermarkets.

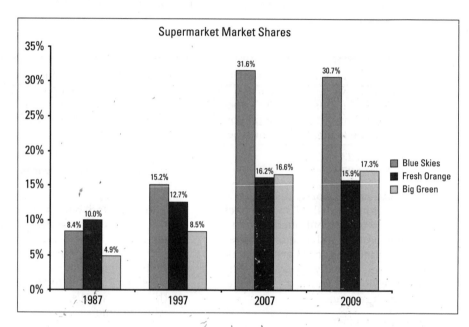

Supermarket Market Shares

21. In 1997, what was the approximate ratio of Blue Skies' market share to that of Big Green?

    (A) 3:2   (B) 9:5   (C) 17:10
    (D) 19:10   (E) 2:1

22. Which of the following statements is supported by the information in the chart?

    A. Blue Skies' market share is steadily increasing.

    B. Big Green's market share is steadily falling.

    C. The three supermarkets in the chart have taken an ever-increasing share of the overall market.

    D. The combined market share of the three supermarkets suffered a fall in 2009.

    E. Discount grocers are responsible for Blue Skies' market share fall in 2009 relative to 2007.

23. Total grocery sales in the UK are approximately £125 billion per year. Roughly how much of that did Big Green take in 2009?

    (A) £6.1 billion   (B) £10.6 billion
    (C) £20.8 billion   (D) £21.6 billion
    (E) £38.4 billon

24. What was the range in market share between the three supermarkets in 1997?

    (A) 6.7%   (B) 14.8%   (C) 15%
    (D) 15.4%   (E) 26.7%

Keeping the Lights on

Catherine is looking to find a new electricity provider and has narrowed down her choice to Midlands Energy and Isis Energy. Their tariffs are shown in the tables below. Electricity usage is measured in pence per kilowatt hour (kWh). A month is thirty days, and a quarter is 90 days.

Midlands Energy Electricity Costs

Energy Package	Cost Per kWh	Daily Standing Charge
Quarterly billing	3.81p	29.97p
Monthly direct debit	3.59p	29.92p

Isis Energy Electricity Costs

Isis Energy Cheapest Package	Peak Cost Per kWh	Off-Peak Cost per kWh	Daily Standing Charge
Domestic economy	15.01p	7.12p	25.56p

25. Assuming that Catherine uses 12 kWh per day, how much more would it cost her per month using Midlands Energy's quarterly billing than its monthly direct debit option?

(A) £0.80   (B) £0.81   (C) £21.90
(D) £22.71   (E) £44.61

26. Of her daily usage of 12 kWh, one-third of Catherine's use is off peak. How much would her total cost per month be with Isis Energy?

(A) £7.67   (B) £8.54   (C) £36.02
(D) £44.56   (E) £52.24

27. If Catherine reduced her electricity usage by 20 per cent, and at the same time switched her consumption pattern to 60 per cent off peak, what would it cost her with Isis Energy's package?

(A) £12.30   (B) £17.29   (C) £37.26
(D) £44.66   (E) £55.23

28. Which of the following statements is false?

A. For Midlands Energy, quarterly billing is more expensive than monthly billing under all circumstances.

B. Isis Energy is cheaper than Midlands Energy's quarterly billing if Catherine's entire monthly energy consumption is less than 18 kWh off peak.

C. If Catherine uses 200 kWh per month, Isis Energy can undercut Midlands Energy's price.

D. Even if Catherine increases her usage to 14 kWh, she will still find it cheaper to use Midlands Energy rather than Isis Energy.

E. Isis Energy's domestic economy package is least cost-effective for very heavy peak users.

Three Score and Ten

The UK Government collects statistics on the life expectancy at birth of people in different parts of the country. The following table contains data for various English regions, segregated by gender.

Life Expectancy at Birth in Years		
Region	*Males*	*Females*
North East	75.8	80.1
North West	75.7	80.3
Yorkshire and the Humber	76.6	81.0
East Midlands	77.3	81.3
West Midlands	76.6	81.1
East of England	78.3	82.3
London	77.4	82.0
South East	78.5	82.4
South West	78.5	82.7

29. What's the range of life expectancy in years between men and women, across England?

   (A) 4.2   (B) 4.3   (C) 4.6
   (D) 7   (E) 8.4

30. What's the approximate average life expectancy in years for women across the English regions? You may assume that each region contributes equally to the average.

   (A) 77.2   (B) 77.3   (C) 81.1
   (D) 81.4   (E) 81.5

31. Expressed as a percentage, how much longer do women live than men in London?

   (A) 5.1%   (B) 5.6%   (C) 5.9%
   (D) 6.2%   (E) 6.5%

32. Which of the following statements is true?

   A. On average, men live longer than women.

   B. A man born in the South West will, on average, live a longer life than a man born in the North East.

   C. The regional variation in life expectancy is greater for women than for men.

   D. A woman born in the North East will, on average, die before a man in the South West who was born on the same day.

   E. The gender difference in life expectancy is least in the West Midlands.

Bottle Bank

George wants to convert his basement into a wine cellar. In order to do this, he needs to add various racks and shelves. The basic dimensions of the room are depicted in the figure below.

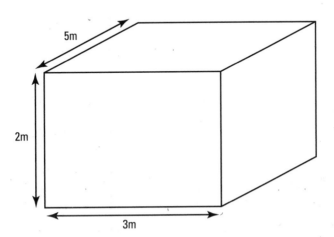

33. George wants to line one long wall with wine racks. The rack is a modular system, with each module 85 cm in height and 120 cm in length and containing up to 72 bottles. How many bottles can he store in the racks if he lines the wall with as many racks as possible?

(A) 72   (B) 144   (C) 288
(D) 576   (E) 706

34. Each module costs £120 excluding VAT. How much does it cost George to line the long wall with as many racks as possible? The rate of VAT is 20 per cent.

(A) £576   (B) £960   (C) £1,152
(D) £1,177   (E) £1,412

35. As well as the racks, George installs a climate control system for the wine cellar. This system costs him a total of £550 to buy and install. Electricity costs are a further 6,600 kWh per year, at a cost of 5p per kWh. Assuming that the capital purchase installation costs are amortised over a ten-year period, how much does it cost George to run the climate control system for a year?

(A) £330   (B) £385   (C) £715
(D) £3,300   (E) £3,850

36. George buys six cases of wine to celebrate the completion of his new cellar. Cases contain a dozen bottles each. He buys three cases of Alsatian Gewürztraminer at £26 per bottle, two cases of Hermitage at £720 per case and a case of fine Bordeaux at £99 per bottle. How much would it cost him to fill his new cellar, at the same average cost per bottle and including these bottles?

(A) £2,254   (B) £3,564   (C) £12,936
(D) £28,512   (E) £155,232

Abstract Reasoning

1. Which figure completes the series?

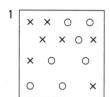

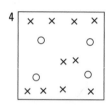

2. Which figure completes the series?

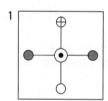

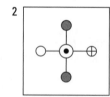

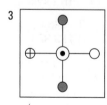

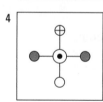

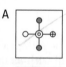

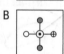

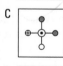

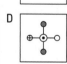

3. Which of the following belongs to Set A?

Set A

Set B

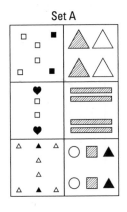
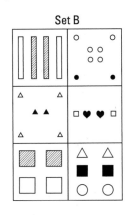
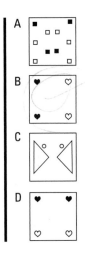

4. Which of the following belongs to Set B?

Set A

Set B

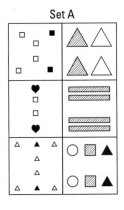
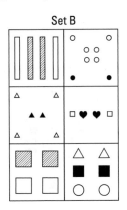

5. Which figure completes the series?

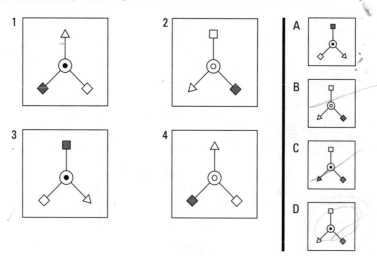

To which set, if either, does each of the test shapes (Q6 to Q10) belong?

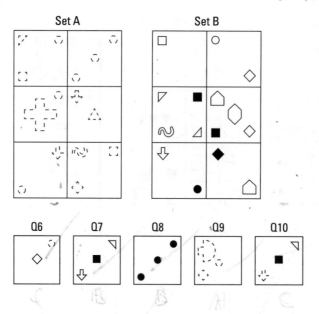

To which set, if either, does each of the test shapes (Q11 to Q15) belong?

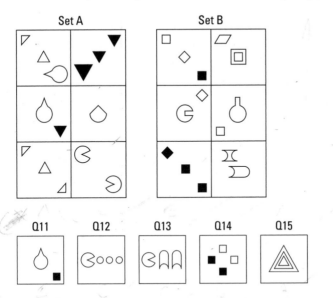

To which set, if either, does each of the test shapes (Q16 to Q20) belong?

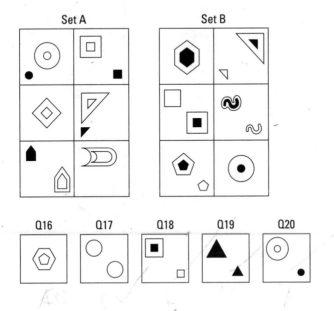

21. Which figure completes the statement?

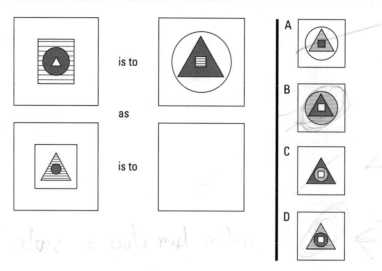

22. Which figure completes the statement?

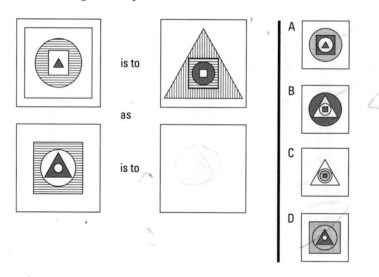

23. Which figure completes the statement?

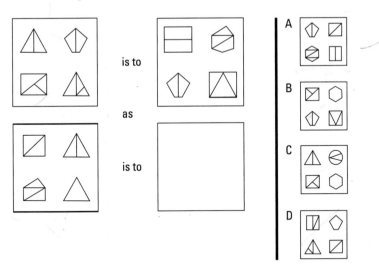

24. Which figure completes the statement?

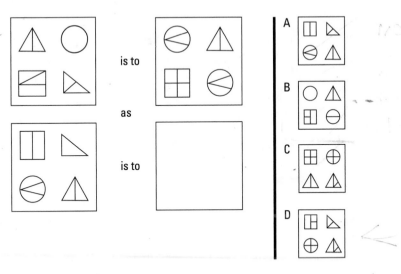

25. Which figure completes the series?

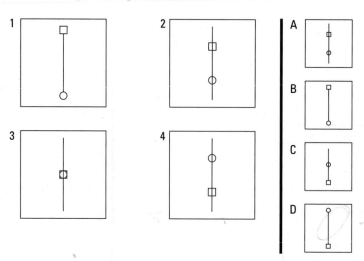

To which set, if either, does each of the test shapes (Q26 to Q30) belong?

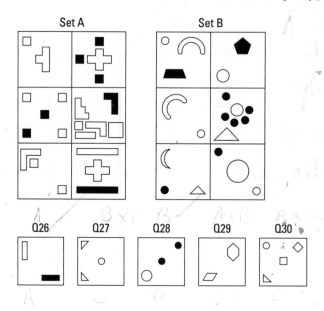

To which set, if either, does each of the test shapes (Q31 to Q35) belong?

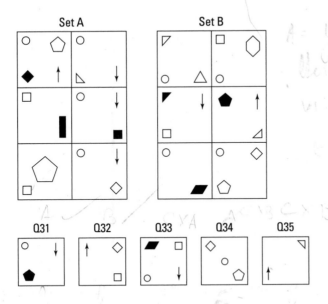

Set A   Set B

Q31   Q32   Q33   Q34   Q35

36. Which figure completes the series?

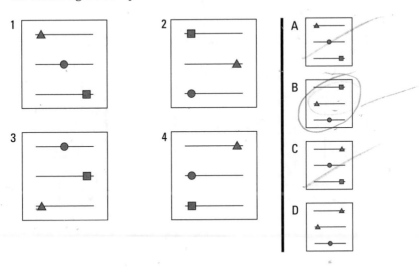

37. Which figure completes the series?

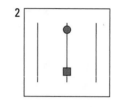

1

3

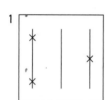

2

4

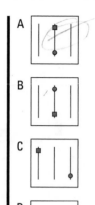

A

B

C

D

38. Which figure completes the series?

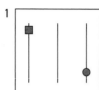

1

3

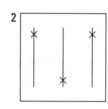

2

4

A

B

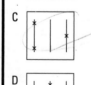

C

D

39. Which figure completes the statement?

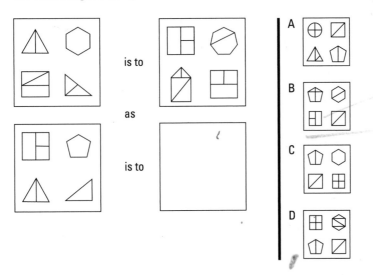

40. Which figure completes the statement?

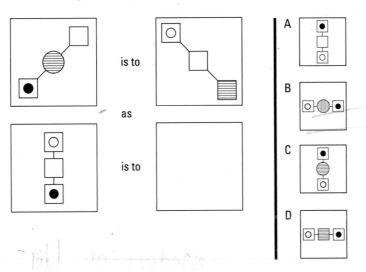

To which set, if either, does each of the test shapes (Q41 to Q45) belong?

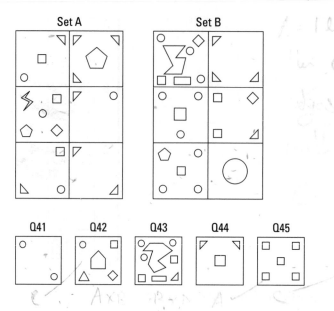

46. Which figure completes the statement?

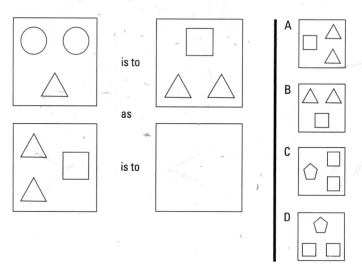

47. Which of the following belongs to Set A?

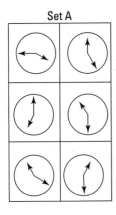

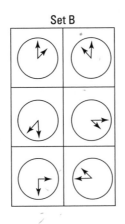

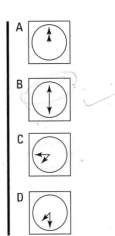

48. Which of the following belongs to Set B?

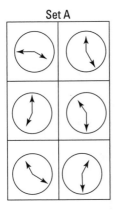

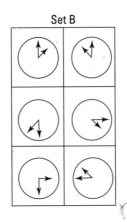

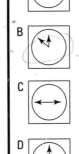

49. Which figure completes the statement?

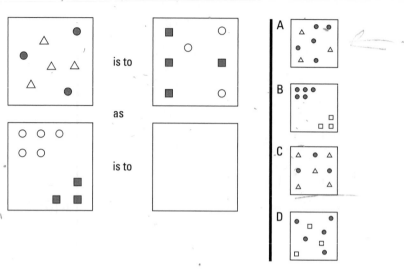

50. Which figure completes the statement?

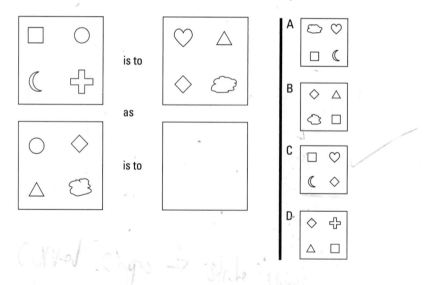

To which set, if either, does each of the test shapes (Q51 to Q55) belong?

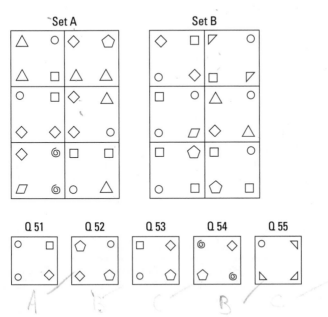

Decision Analysis

Scenario

Football Games

The intemperate manager of Cannons United has been banished from the dugout for swearing repeatedly at match officials. Prohibited from talking to his players, he's forced to communicate surreptitiously by passing written messages to his assistant manager down at the side lines. To prevent the Football Association from accusing him of communicating with his team from the stands, the manager uses a complex code. This table shows the manager's code.

The Manager's Code

The Players	The Pitch	Movements	Types
Defender = ◀	Net = ^	Fast = ʊ	Increase = ⇉
Midfielder = △	Goalposts = ⌣	Slow = ʊ	Decrease = ⇇
Striker = ▶	Penalty Spot = ⁝	Attack = →	Talk = ⇆
Keeper = ▽	Halfway Line = ‡	Defend = ←	Walk = ↔
Cannons = ▲	Corner = ↖	Score = ☗	Approve = ↘
Opponent = ▼	Whistle = ⌣	Shoot = ↯	Disapprove = ⌢
Referee = ↻	Hand = ⊢	Pass = ↳	
Ball = ▛	Head = →⊦		

You're the assistant manager, communicating via code with your unhappy boss sitting in the stands. Your boss depends on your help to change the course of the game.

1. What is the best interpretation of the following coded message?

▼, ↪, ▶

A. Pass the ball to the defender.
B. Pass the ball to the striker.
C. Pass the ball to the midfielder.
D. Pass the ball to the keeper.
E. The striker should shoot.

2. What is the best interpretation of the following coded message?

↪, △, ↪, ▶, ⚡

A. Pass from midfield to striker then shoot.
B. Pass from defence to the striker then shoot.
C. Pass to midfield then to the striker then shoot.
D. Shoot frequently from midfield and from the striker.
E. Move midfield into attack and shoot.

3. What is the best interpretation of the following coded message?

⇉(▲, ↪, ▼, ▲)

A. Move the ball around near the opposition's goal.
B. Attack a lot.
C. Stay in defence.
D. Don't attack.
E. Keep possession.

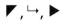

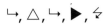

4. What is the best interpretation of the following coded message?

⇉ ⌃, ↻

A. The referee will blow his whistle soon.
B. The referee should book the opposition.
C. The referee will book our player.
D. The referee's an idiot.
E. The referee can be bribed.

5. What is the best interpretation of the following coded message?

↻, ⌣, ⇉(⌃ ⇆), ▼

A. Send off that opposition player, referee!
B. Substitute our player.
C. Tell the referee we're going to make a substitution.
D. The opposition is telling the referee it's substituting a player.
E. The opposition is trying to get our players sent off.

6. What is the best interpretation of the following coded message?

◀◀(⌣), ←↖

A. Tell the defence to press forwards after this corner.
B. Two defenders should run from the goalposts in order to defend this corner.
C. I want one of the defenders to take this corner.
D. I don't like the way the defence keeps hanging back near the goalposts on corners.
E. I want two defenders to stay near the goalposts to defend this corner.

7. What is the best interpretation of the following coded message?

$$(\triangle \triangle), \rightarrow \circlearrowleft$$

   A. The midfield is running too fast.
   B. The midfielders will get exhausted.
   C. Midfield needs to attack faster.
   D. I'm going to tell off the midfield for running too much.
   E. Tell the midfield to run back and support the defence.

8. What is the best interpretation of the following coded message?

$$(\blacktriangle \text{⇧}) \rightrightarrows, \blacktriangledown \text{⇧}$$

   A. We need to score one more than the opposition does.
   B. The opposition scored more than we did.
   C. Score now, quickly, while the opposition is attacking.
   D. Don't pass; shoot and score!
   E. We're getting better now that the opposition has scored.

9. What is the best interpretation of the following coded message?

$$\circlearrowright, \blacktriangledown \blacktriangleleft, \vdash \blacktriangledown$$

   A. Referee, that was a clear handball by the opposition.
   B. Referee, the opposing defender handballed!
   C. Tell the referee to get his hand out of his pocket and book the opposition for handball.
   D. I don't want the referee to see us handball while defending.
   E. Tell the defence to handball, but distract the referee first.

10. What is the best interpretation of the following coded message?

$$\text{⚡}\blacktriangledown, \wedge, (\text{⌒} \rightrightarrows) \blacktriangleright$$

   A. I hate the way you shoot.
   B. Just score!
   C. Tell that idiot striker to just hit the ball into the net!
   D. Don't keep passing it around so much.
   E. That was a bad shot.

11. What is the best interpretation of the following coded message?

$$\blacktriangleright \text{⚡}, \triangledown \leftarrow, \triangle \text{⇧}$$

   A. The keeper let the striker and midfielder score.
   B. The keeper tried to defend the midfielder's shot, letting the striker score.
   C. The striker took a shot at the defending goalkeeper after the midfielder scored.
   D. The striker didn't score, but the midfielder did.
   E. The keeper saved from the striker, but the midfielder scored on the rebound.

12. Translate the following into the manager's code:

Tell me if you want me to substitute a striker for a defender.

   A. $\leftrightarrows, (\leftrightarrows \leftrightarrow) \blacktriangleright, \blacktriangleleft$
   B. $\leftrightarrows, \blacktriangleright, \blacktriangleleft$
   C. $(\leftrightarrows \leftrightarrow) \blacktriangleright, \blacktriangleleft$
   D. $\leftrightarrows, (\leftrightarrows \leftrightarrow) \blacktriangleleft, \blacktriangleright$
   E. $\leftrightarrows, \leftrightarrows (\blacktriangleright), \blacktriangleleft$

13. What is the best interpretation of the following coded message?

    ↺ ↔, ▼ ‡

    A. I want you all to attack now.
    B. Shoot from where you are, quickly!
    C. Pull everyone back into our own half to defend.
    D. Run into the opposition's half.
    E. Press forward into the opposition's half, slowly.

14. What is the best interpretation of the following coded message?

    (⇧ ⇧)(‿‡)

    A. Score twice in each half.
    B. Score a goal in either half.
    C. Score two goals in this half.
    D. Scoring twice will win this match.
    E. This match is a rematch.

15. Translate the following into the manager's code:

    Place the ball on the corner spot and score when the referee blows his whistle.

    A. ▼↖, ↻‿, ⇧

    B. ▼↖, ⇧, ↻‿

    C. ↻‿, ⇧, ▼↖

    D. ↻, ▼↖, ⇧

    E. ⇧▼, ‿

16. What is the best interpretation of the following coded message?

    (△△)↦ ▶, →ı ⇧

    A. Tell the striker to head the ball into the net.
    B. Midfield needs to pass up to the striker so he can head a goal.
    C. The midfield are passing among themselves too much; give it to the striker so he can head the ball and score.
    D. Pass quickly to the striker so he can head the ball into the goal.
    E. Don't pass the ball to the striker, midfield; head it to him so he can score.

17. What is the best interpretation of the following coded message?

    ▲(⇉(↔↻)↦), ▶▶

    A. We need to pass the ball faster through the team, up to the strikers.
    B. More passing, more speed.
    C. I need us pushing further up the pitch and getting the ball to the strikers.
    D. I need everyone to run faster, pass more and get the ball to the strikers.
    E. Tell the strikers to hold the ball up and move more quickly.

18. What is the best interpretation of the following coded message?

↘▲, ⇉→

A. Congratulations, you won!
B. Don't wait for my approval, just attack!
C. Stop attacking, you've done what you needed to.
D. The attack's going well.
E. Well done, lads; now attack, attack, attack!

19. What is the best interpretation of the following coded message?

↻⇉(↻‿), ⇉←

A. Tell the referee to blow his whistle; we can't defend any longer.
B. The referee will blow his whistle any minute now; hang on!
C. Our defence is begging the referee to blow his whistle.
D. The referee is helping our defence with his interruptions of the game.
E. The referee has lost his whistle while running into defence.

20. What is the best interpretation of the following coded message?

▲(◀◀), ↻⇉

A. We need our defence to slow the game down.
B. Our defence have to speed the game up.
C. Their defenders are playing too slowly.
D. Their defenders are wasting time by talking to each other.
E. Break their defence quickly to end the game.

21. What is the best interpretation of the following coded message?

⇆, ▲(△△), →(↦↦), ▲(▶▶)

A. We need our strikers to drop back and pass from midfield.
B. Our midfield aren't making enough attacking crosses to attack.
C. Get our midfield to send more penetrating crosses to the strikers.
D. If our midfield can attack more, we'll get more corners.
E. The midfield are passing to themselves too much, and not attacking.

22. What is the best interpretation of the following coded message?

▼▼, ⇆, ↻, (‿⌒)↔, ◀

A. The opposition players won't stop talking to the referee about our defender.
B. The referee's trying to decide whether to send off our defender.
C. Our defender managed to get the referee to send off the opposition's striker.
D. The opponents managed to get our defender sent off.
E. The opponents managed to get the referee to send our defender off the pitch.

23. Which **two** of the following terms would be the most useful additions to the code if you had to translate the following message?

If you don't start playing better, our owners are going to sell the lot of you.

A. Play

B. Match

C. Owner

D. Sell

E. Lot

24. Which **two** of the following terms would be the most useful additions to the code if you had to translate the following message?

I'm over the moon, but we'll still take each match as it comes and give 110 per cent.

A. Match

B. Moon

C. Over

D. Calm

E. 110%

25. What is the best interpretation of the following coded message?

▲◀(↖⏝), (▲◀▽)←⌃

A. Get one of our defenders to cover the goalpost nearest the corner, and another to stand next to the keeper and block the net.

B. Get our defenders near the goalposts and the keeper in front of the net.

C. Get one of our defenders on that corner spot and the other with the keeper in front of the net.

D. Get the defenders around the corner taker, and place the keeper in front of the net.

E. I want one defender on the nearside goalpost and the other out by the penalty spot.

26. What is the best interpretation of the following coded message?

↻⇉(↺⏝), ▲↖, ⇑

A. Take the corner and score.

B. Force the corner by kicking the ball into touch in the last minute.

C. It's the last minute of the match, we have a corner . . . and score!

D. Score from this corner and we take the lead.

E. We need a last-minute corner.

27. What is the best interpretation of the following coded message?

↳,▶,→ı,⚡

A. Pass to the striker to score with his head.

B. Pass to the defender to score with his head.

C. Pass to the striker to shoot with his head.

D. Pass to the defender to score with his head.

E. Pass to the keeper to stop with his hands.

28. What is the best interpretation of the following coded message?

A. The striker doesn't want to shoot the penalty.

B. The captain disapproves of the penalty shot.

C. The striker scored from the penalty spot.

D. Unfortunately, the striker scored the penalty.

E. The striker's unhappy about the penalty point.

Situational Judgement Test

Chiti Patel, a 35-year-old woman, walks into A&E with two broken ribs and bruises on both arms and one side of her neck. She insists that she's fallen down the stairs, but Dr Osode, the A&E registrar, suspects that she may be the victim of domestic abuse.

How **appropriate** are each of the following responses by **Dr Osode** in this situation?

1. Treat Mrs Patel for her injuries and leave it at that.

   A. A very appropriate thing to do.
   B. Appropriate, but not ideal.
   C. Inappropriate, but not awful.
   D. A very inappropriate thing to do.

2. Explore Mrs Patel's home situation.

   A. A very appropriate thing to do.
   B. Appropriate, but not ideal.
   C. Inappropriate, but not awful.
   D. A very inappropriate thing to do.

3. Encourage Mrs Patel to seek help if she needs it.

   A. A very appropriate thing to do.
   B. Appropriate, but not ideal.
   C. Inappropriate, but not awful.
   D. A very inappropriate thing to do.

4. Treat Mrs Patel for her injuries and then report her husband to the police.

   A. A very appropriate thing to do.
   B. Appropriate, but not ideal.
   C. Inappropriate, but not awful.
   D. A very inappropriate thing to do.

5. Establish whether any children or vulnerable adults live with Mrs Patel.

   A. A very appropriate thing to do.
   B. Appropriate, but not ideal.
   C. Inappropriate, but not awful.
   D. A very inappropriate thing to do.

6. Document his full conversation with Mrs Patel.

   A. A very appropriate thing to do.
   B. Appropriate, but not ideal.
   C. Inappropriate, but not awful.
   D. A very inappropriate thing to do.

Six months later, Dr Osode bumps into Chiti Patel in a supermarket. Mrs Patel tells him that she's left her abusive relationship and is currently receiving counselling. She invites Dr Osode to dine in her favourite restaurant to thank him for his help.

How **appropriate** are each of the following responses by **Dr Osode** in this situation?

7. Accept the invitation, because Chiti Patel's no longer his patient.

   A. A very appropriate thing to do.
   B. Appropriate, but not ideal.
   C. Inappropriate, but not awful.
   D. A very inappropriate thing to do.

8. Accept the invitation, but insist on paying for his dinner.

   A. A very appropriate thing to do.
   B. Appropriate, but not ideal.
   C. Inappropriate, but not awful.
   D. A very inappropriate thing to do.

9. Politely decline her invitation.

   A. A very appropriate thing to do.
   B. Appropriate, but not ideal.
   C. Inappropriate, but not awful.
   D. A very inappropriate thing to do.

10. Offer to buy Mrs Patel a drink instead.

   A. A very appropriate thing to do.
   B. Appropriate, but not ideal.
   C. Inappropriate, but not awful.
   D. A very inappropriate thing to do.

Mr Glover, a middle-aged patient on the gastrointestinal ward, has been diagnosed with pancreatic cancer. The gastrointestinal consultant asks Marisa, a foundation year 1 (FY1) doctor, to break the bad news to Emma Glover, the patient's daughter. Marisa calls Emma to the hospital and meets her at the main reception. 'How is my father?' asks Emma, looking visibly anxious.

How **important** to take into account are the following considerations for **Marisa** when deciding how to respond to the situation?

11. The setting of their conversation.

    A. Very important.

    B. Important.

    C. Of minor importance.

    D. Not important at all.

12. How much Emma already knows about her father's condition.

    A. Very important.

    B. Important.

    C. Of minor importance.

    D. Not important at all.

13. Whether Emma feels close to her father.

    A. Very important.

    B. Important.

    C. Of minor importance.

    D. Not important at all.

14. Mr Glover's confidentiality.

    A. Very important.

    B. Important.

    C. Of minor importance.

    D. Not important at all.

Mr Firkin is a 78-year-old man with a history of memory problems. He's recently developed a chest pain that keeps him up at night. He presents to his GP surgery accompanied by his daughter, Amanda. The GP, Dr Jamal, would like to refer Mr Firkin to a specialist, but Mr Firkin's adamant that he doesn't want to go to hospital. Amanda, who's very worried about her father, asks Dr Jamal to refer him anyway, because he 'no longer has all his mind'.

How **important** to take into account are the following considerations for **Dr Jamal** when deciding how to respond to the situation?

15. Mr Firkin's degree of capacity to decide about his care.

A. Very important.

B. Important.

C. Of minor importance.

D. Not important at all.

16. The fact that Mr Firkin has recently been diagnosed with a form of dementia.

A. Very important.

B. Important.

C. Of minor importance.

D. Not important at all.

17. The severity and likely cause or causes of Mr Firkin's chest pain.

A. Very important.

B. Important.

C. Of minor importance.

D. Not important at all.

18. Amanda's degree of concern for her father.

A. Very important.

B. Important.

C. Of minor importance.

D. Not important at all.

The second-year medical students have been divided into groups of six to work on a poster presentation for their public health module. Liz has been assigned to the group responsible for the smoking ban. However, the other students are concerned that she's not pulling her weight.

How **appropriate** are each of the following responses by **the other students in the group** in this situation?

19. Speak to Liz as a group.

A. A very appropriate thing to do.

B. Appropriate, but not ideal.

C. Inappropriate, but not awful.

D. A very inappropriate thing to do.

20. Nominate one of the students to speak with Liz in private.

A. A very appropriate thing to do.

B. Appropriate, but not ideal.

C. Inappropriate, but not awful.

D. A very inappropriate thing to do.

21. Do nothing, because the project is advancing well anyway.

A. A very appropriate thing to do.

B. Appropriate, but not ideal.

C. Inappropriate, but not awful.

D. A very inappropriate thing to do.

22. Discuss the issue with the course leader.

A. A very appropriate thing to do.

B. Appropriate, but not ideal.

C. Inappropriate, but not awful.

D. A very inappropriate thing to do.

A 5-year-old has developed a rash and fever and is vomiting profusely. When the consultant paediatrician tries to examine his abdomen, he starts crying and screaming that he wants to go home.

How **appropriate** are each of the following responses by **the consultant paediatrician** in this situation?

23. Carry on with the examination, because the child's very ill.

    A. A very appropriate thing to do.
    B. Appropriate, but not ideal.
    C. Inappropriate, but not awful.
    D. A very inappropriate thing to do.

24. Ask the boy's mother to reassure him and hold his hand.

    A. A very appropriate thing to do.
    B. Appropriate, but not ideal.
    C. Inappropriate, but not awful.
    D. A very inappropriate thing to do.

25. Give up the examination and rely on the history alone.

    A. A very appropriate thing to do.
    B. Appropriate, but not ideal.
    C. Inappropriate, but not awful.
    D. A very inappropriate thing to do.

26. Attend to other patients and return in a couple of hours.

    A. A very appropriate thing to do.
    B. Appropriate, but not ideal.
    C. Inappropriate, but not awful.
    D. A very inappropriate thing to do.

Linda, a FY1 doctor who's just started work, is having a lot of trouble inserting a cannula into an elderly patient's veins. She's tried on three separate occasions, and on the third occasion the patient screamed out in pain.

How **important** to take into account are the following considerations for **Linda** when deciding how to respond to the situation?

27. Her fear of disappointing her consultant.

    A. Very important.

    B. Important.

    C. Of minor importance.

    D. Not important at all.

28. Her desire to get more practice inserting cannulas.

    A. Very important.

    B. Important.

    C. Of minor importance.

    D. Not important at all.

29. The clinical need for a cannula.

    A. Very important.

    B. Important.

    C. Of minor importance.

    D. Not important at all.

30. The patient's distress.

    A. Very important.

    B. Important.

    C. Of minor importance.

    D. Not important at all.

Angelina, a final-year medical student, is on her A&E attachment. It's a very busy shift and all the doctors are working flat out. Mr Jones is angry, because he's been waiting almost six hours to be seen. One of the doctors asks Angelina to go and speak to Mr Jones.

How **appropriate** are each of the following responses by **Angelina** in this situation?

31. Tell Mr Jones that his behaviour is inappropriate and selfish.

A. A very appropriate thing to do.
B. Appropriate, but not ideal.
C. Inappropriate, but not awful.
D. A very inappropriate thing to do.

32. Promise Mr Jones that he'll be seen next.

A. A very appropriate thing to do.
B. Appropriate, but not ideal.
C. Inappropriate, but not awful.
D. A very inappropriate thing to do.

33. Apologise to Mr Jones and blame the situation on the Government and hospital management.

A. A very appropriate thing to do.
B. Appropriate, but not ideal.
C. Inappropriate, but not awful.
D. A very inappropriate thing to do.

34. Apologise to Mr Jones, explaining that the doctors are all very busy and that he'll be seen as soon as possible.

A. A very appropriate thing to do.
B. Appropriate, but not ideal.
C. Inappropriate, but not awful.
D. A very inappropriate thing to do.

The third-year medical students are on their lunch break. Laura sits at a table with Luke and four other medical students. As they eat, Luke begins cracking jokes at the expense of some of the patients in the cancer unit.

How **appropriate** are each of the following responses by **Laura** in this situation?

35. Subtly change the subject.

A. A very appropriate thing to do.

B. Appropriate, but not ideal.

C. Inappropriate, but not awful.

D. A very inappropriate thing to do.

36. Do nothing, reasoning that no real harm's being done.

A. A very appropriate thing to do.

B. Appropriate, but not ideal.

C. Inappropriate, but not awful.

D. A very inappropriate thing to do.

37. Tell Luke in front of the other students to stop making such jokes.

A. A very appropriate thing to do.

B. Appropriate, but not ideal.

C. Inappropriate, but not awful.

D. A very inappropriate thing to do.

38. Take Luke aside and tell him to stop making such jokes.

A. A very appropriate thing to do.

B. Appropriate, but not ideal.

C. Inappropriate, but not awful.

D. A very inappropriate thing to do.

David, an FY1 doctor, is talking to Jess, a 26-year-old woman who is being treated for an overdose. Jess tells David that she'd like to leave the hospital, cheerfully assuring him that she's feeling fine and that the overdose was just one big accident.

How **important** are the following for **David** to take into account when deciding how to respond to the situation?

39. The type and size of the overdose.

    A. Very important.
    B. Important.
    C. Of minor importance.
    D. Not important at all.

40. Jess's mental state.

    A. Very important.
    B. Important.
    C. Of minor importance.
    D. Not important at all.

41. Jess's cheerfulness.

    A. Very important.
    B. Important.
    C. Of minor importance.
    D. Not important at all.

42. The need for a senior or specialist (psychiatric) opinion.

    A. Very important.
    B. Important.
    C. Of minor importance.
    D. Not important at all.

On her second day, Samantha, a newly appointed FY1 doctor, overhears the head nurse complaining about her, telling three other nurses that she's lazy and incompetent and 'already thinks she's better than us'.

How **appropriate** are each of the following responses by **Samantha** in this situation?

43. Say nothing, because doing so would only make things worse.

    A. A very appropriate thing to do.

    B. Appropriate, but not ideal.

    C. Inappropriate, but not awful.

    D. A very inappropriate thing to do.

44. Report the nurse to the hospital authorities.

    A. A very appropriate thing to do.

    B. Appropriate, but not ideal.

    C. Inappropriate, but not awful.

    D. A very inappropriate thing to do.

45. Interrupt the nurse there and then, and tell her that her behaviour's unacceptable.

    A. A very appropriate thing to do.

    B. Appropriate, but not ideal.

    C. Inappropriate, but not awful.

    D. A very inappropriate thing to do.

46. Come back later and have a quiet word with the nurse.

    A. A very appropriate thing to do.

    B. Appropriate, but not ideal.

    C. Inappropriate, but not awful.

    D. A very inappropriate thing to do.

47. Invite some of the nurses out for a drink to improve her standing among them.

    A. A very appropriate thing to do.

    B. Appropriate, but not ideal.

    C. Inappropriate, but not awful.

    D. A very inappropriate thing to do.

Andrew, a fourth-year medical student, is sitting in Mr Kumar's clinic. Mr Kumar, a consultant surgeon, is explaining a procedure to a patient, but Andrew's disappointed by his explanation. In particular, he feels that Mr Kumar ought to have been much more precise and given more detail.

How **appropriate** are each of the following responses by **Andrew** in this situation?

48. Immediately provide the patient with his own fuller explanation of the procedure.

  A. A very appropriate thing to do.
  B. Appropriate, but not ideal.
  C. Inappropriate, but not awful.
  D. A very inappropriate thing to do.

49. Wait until the consultation is finished, and only then provide the patient with his own fuller explanation of the procedure.

  A. A very appropriate thing to do.
  B. Appropriate, but not ideal.
  C. Inappropriate, but not awful.
  D. A very inappropriate thing to do.

50. Wait until the consultation is finished and discuss his feelings with Mr Kumar.

  A. A very appropriate thing to do.
  B. Appropriate, but not ideal.
  C. Inappropriate, but not awful.
  D. A very inappropriate thing to do.

51. Politely ask the medical school to attach him to a different consultant.

  A. A very appropriate thing to do.
  B. Appropriate, but not ideal.
  C. Inappropriate, but not awful.
  D. A very inappropriate thing to do.

Mr Brown attends Dr Stewart's clinic and discovers that he's HIV positive. One month later, his partner, Mr Poole, attends the same clinic and asks for an HIV test. In the course of Dr Stewart and Mr Poole's conversation, Mr Poole says that his partner, Mr Brown, is HIV negative.

How **appropriate** are each of the following responses by **Dr Stewart** in this situation?

52. Tell Mr Poole that Mr Brown is in fact HIV positive.

  A. A very appropriate thing to do.
  B. Appropriate, but not ideal.
  C. Inappropriate, but not awful.
  D. A very inappropriate thing to do.

53. Call Mr Brown and try to persuade him to tell Mr Poole that he is in fact HIV positive.

  A. A very appropriate thing to do.
  B. Appropriate, but not ideal.
  C. Inappropriate, but not awful.
  D. A very inappropriate thing to do.

54. Advise Mr Poole to have protected sex.

  A. A very appropriate thing to do.
  B. Appropriate, but not ideal.
  C. Inappropriate, but not awful.
  D. A very inappropriate thing to do.

55. Respect Mr Brown's confidentiality and do nothing more about it.

  A. A very appropriate thing to do.
  B. Appropriate, but not ideal.
  C. Inappropriate, but not awful.
  D. A very inappropriate thing to do.

Nancy presents to A&E with two broken ribs. She tells the A&E registrar, Dr Sullivan, that her partner beat her and that she's worried that he may do so again. However, she insists on going back home and asks Dr Sullivan not to tell the police or social services about her partner's abusive behaviour.

How **appropriate** are each of the following responses by **Dr Sullivan** in this situation?

56. Insist that Nancy tells the police before providing her with treatment.

A. A very appropriate thing to do.
B. Appropriate, but not ideal.
C. Inappropriate, but not awful.
D. A very inappropriate thing to do.

57. Drop the subject and do nothing more.

A. A very appropriate thing to do.
B. Appropriate, but not ideal.
C. Inappropriate, but not awful.
D. A very inappropriate thing to do.

58. Call the police or social services and report the assault.

A. A very appropriate thing to do.
B. Appropriate, but not ideal.
C. Inappropriate, but not awful.
D. A very inappropriate thing to do.

59. Support Nancy in making a decision in her own best interests.

A. A very appropriate thing to do.
B. Appropriate, but not ideal.
C. Inappropriate, but not awful.
D. A very inappropriate thing to do.

Mr Hawthorne suffers from a heart condition that can no longer be adequately controlled by medication alone. His GP, Dr Tzakanikis, recommends surgery, as do Mr Hawthorne's wife and children. However, Mr Hawthorne is frightened of surgery and reluctant to accept their recommendation. When Dr Tzakanikis offers to refer him to a cardiac surgeon, Mr Hawthorne goes along with it 'because that's what everybody wants'.

How **important** to take into account are the following considerations for **Dr Tzakanikis** when deciding how to respond to the situation?

60. That Mr Hawthorne understands the potential benefits and risks of surgery.

  A. Very important.

  B. Important.

  C. Of minor importance.

  D. Not important at all.

61. That Mr Hawthorne understands the potential benefits and risks of alternatives to surgery, including the option not to treat.

  A. Very important.

  B. Important.

  C. Of minor importance.

  D. Not important at all.

62. That Mr Hawthorne is 81 years old.

  A. Very important.

  B. Important.

  C. Of minor importance.

  D. Not important at all.

63. That Mr Hawthorne doesn't feel pressured into accepting his recommendation.

  A. Very important.

  B. Important.

  C. Of minor importance.

  D. Not important at all.

Mrs Gosford is an 88-year-old in-patient with terminal cancer. Dr Banerjee, one of the junior doctors, is keen to ensure that Mrs Gosford dies in a dignified and peaceful manner, so he asks Dr Rauch, the consultant, to make and record a decision not to attempt cardiopulmonary resuscitation (CPR).

How **important** to take into account are the following considerations for **Dr Rauch** when deciding how to respond to the situation?

64. Dr Banerjee's motives for requesting a 'do not attempt CPR' order.

A. Very important.
B. Important.
C. Of minor importance.
D. Not important at all.

65. Mrs Gosford's age.

A. Very important.
B. Important.
C. Of minor importance.
D. Not important at all.

66. Mrs Gosford's opinion on the matter.

A. Very important.
B. Important.
C. Of minor importance.
D. Not important at all.

67. The opinion of the nursing staff.

A. Very important.
B. Important.
C. Of minor importance.
D. Not important at all.

Clive is taken to A&E with a stab wound. Clive insists that the stab wound is self-inflicted. However, Dr Ochoa, the A&E junior doctor, suspects that he's lying from fear of the gang that attacked him. She considers contacting the police to report the stab wound.

How **important** to take into account are the following considerations for **Dr Ochoa** when deciding how to respond to the situation?

68. The depth of the stab wound.

    A. Very important.

    B. Important.

    C. Of minor importance.

    D. Not important at all.

69. The public interest.

    A. Very important.

    B. Important.

    C. Of minor importance.

    D. Not important at all.

70. The prevention, detection or prosecution of a serious crime.

    A. Very important.

    B. Important.

    C. Of minor importance.

    D. Not important at all.

71. Clive's fear.

    A. Very important.

    B. Important.

    C. Of minor importance.

    D. Not important at all.

Chapter 12

Practice Test Two: Answers and Explanations

In This Chapter

▶ Answering the questions in Practice Test Two

▶ Understanding the answers

Verbal Reasoning

1. A: True

   This answer follows logically from the information in the first paragraph. You know that the Sun crosses the observer's meridian at noon – the Sun is no longer east or west of you. If the Sun is neither east nor west, it must be south or north (or, rarely, directly overhead). You also know that when the Sun's at this point, the celestial meridian corresponds to your longitude.

2. A: True

   The first two paragraphs together tell you that you can calculate both longitude and latitude at noon. You also know that finding longitude and latitude is a cornerstone of the navigator's day. From this you can deduce that the noon sighting of the sun is important to navigators.

3. B: False

   You know that the Sun's at your zenith when it's directly above you. When the Sun's directly beneath you (on the opposite side of the Earth), the Sun is at your nadir – but you don't need to know this to answer the question.

4. C: Can't tell

You know only that the Sun appears to travel around the Earth. The passage doesn't say whether the Earth revolves around the Sun.

Don't bring in outside knowledge when answering questions in the verbal reasoning subtest.

5. A: True

On hearing the music, the author immediately recognised the advert as being for Marks & Spencer. Thus, brand awareness is reinforced.

Marks & Spencer isn't the only company to recognise the usefulness of a catchy soundtrack, although we think that their choice of tune is a lot more melodious than the offerings from certain other companies.

6. C: Can't tell

Just because the chocolate pudding campaign worked on Claire doesn't necessarily mean that Claire's in the target demographic or that Claire's demographic is important in all advertising campaigns.

Beware when reasoning from the specific to the general in the verbal reasoning subtest. Such logic can lead you to draw conclusions that the text doesn't necessarily support.

7. C: Can't tell

You know that pudding sales rose by 288 per cent, but you don't know about the overall increase in food sales.

8. A: True

The overall tone of the passage is that of someone impressed by the advertising, from the enthusiastic description of the commercial itself to the specific sentence that he found it inspirational, and the exclamation mark at the end of the passage.

9. B: True

The passage is quite clear in its statement that Cowell has more autonomy than do most people in the music industry.

10. A: True

Cowell is metaphorically described as laying golden eggs for Sony.

11. B: False

The passage documents failures in Cowell's early career.

12. A: True

The author explains Cowell's relationship with Sony as being a case of enlightened self-interest. He also says that Cowell has more autonomy within that relationship than most people have in the music industry. Therefore, in the author's opinion, enlightened self-interest underpins that relative autonomy.

13. A: True

Although not all ethnic groups are immigrant groups, the passage says that sociologists interested in ethnicity study immigration, and it talks about immigrant groups as being from different cultures, countries and traditions to those of the host country.

14. C: Can't tell

The passage cites the search for work as one reason why immigration into the US in the early 20th century was concentrated in the major cities, but the text doesn't exclude other causes of immigration.

15. A: True

The passage defines assimilation alternatively as a great melting pot and as immigrants adopting the language and traditions of their new community.

16. C: Can't tell

The passage says that this is the case if the theory of assimilation is correct – but does not go so far as to say that it is.

17. A: True

The passage states this clearly.

18. B: False

Ackerman plans to diversify the portfolio of shows that Fresh One makes, which means that Ackerman plans to have fewer shows centred around Oliver and more shows centred on other things.

19. A: True

The passage says that they can make businesses more sustainable and saleable. Doing so would have the potential to increase a business owner's wealth.

20. C: Can't tell

    This was David Page's plan, but the passage doesn't tell you whether the plan was well realised.

21. C: Can't tell

    The passage tells you that most broadcasts will be viewed on 'tablets and iPads', but the text doesn't give the relative popularity of each. Therefore, you can't tell whether the iPad subset alone will represent a majority of viewers.

    At the time of writing, iPads are the most popular tablet device, but you can't use outside knowledge to answer the question.

22. A: True

    The passage cites this as one of the three reasons behind the shift.

23. A: True

    The passage notes that online viewership is increasing faster than online advertising revenue.

24. C: Can't tell

    This statement may well be correct, but the passage doesn't commit to this outcome. In fact, other factors may intervene to prevent digital eyeballs being worth as much as TV eyeballs to advertisers. For example, the demographic or people's attention to advertising may differ.

25. B: False

    Sun Tzu suggests the opposite, using the opponent's strength in one position against him and attacking elsewhere instead. A less martial analogy is to think about how to negotiate with someone: if the other person is fixated by one particular issue, it can be helpful to compromise on something else before returning to discuss the issue.

26. A: True

    Sun Tzu repeatedly returns to this theme of speed being crucial to successful warfare, in particular when he says 'the enemy cannot pursue, because we retire too quickly'. Similarly, speed of action is often crucial in making the most of your opportunities, otherwise someone else gets there first and exploits those opportunities.

27. C: Can't tell

    The passage doesn't make this assertion. However, the explanations of answers 25 and 26 show that this can be the case.

28. A: True

   This statement is the overriding message of the passage and is spelt out in the last paragraph.

29. D: A blazing fire is in front of a ramp with a low wall.

   The blazing fire is *behind* a ramp with a low wall. The prisoners must be accustomed to darkness, since 'When a prisoner is unshackled and turned towards the fire, he suffers sharp pains, but after some time his eyes accommodate to the light' (A). The back of the cave is indeed like a screen onto which the shadows of the statues are reflected, since 'the fire casts the shadows of the statues onto the back of the cave' (B). The prisoners must be unaware of what's going on behind them, since 'As the prisoners only ever see the shadows, they naturally come to believe that the shadows are the objects themselves' (C).

30. A: The prisoners are reluctant to leave the cave.

   The prisoners must be 'dragged out of the cave', which means that they're reluctant (A), not keen (B), to leave the cave. However likely C and D may seem, they can't be inferred from the text.

31. C: Education is a matter of learning facts.

   The final sentence says 'the purpose of education is to drag the prisoner as far out of the cave as possible, not to show him this or that particular object, but to turn his whole soul towards the sun.' In other words, the author's more likely to believe that education's a matter of seeing more clearly (D) than of learning isolated facts. The shadows on the back of the cave are shadows of statues, so they're shadows of replicas rather than of real objects (A). Given that the state of the prisoner within the cave is one of shackled ignorance, it stands to reason that a prisoner who's managed to leave the cave is unlikely to want to return (B).

32. D: An allegory

   A story (A) is an account or recital of an event or a series of events, either true or fictitious. A myth (B) is a traditional story dealing with supernatural beings, ancestors or heroes that serves as a foundation for the identity, aspirations and culture of a people. A fable (C) is a narrative, usually short, with an edifying or cautionary moral, and often employing animals that speak and act like humans. An allegory is the embodiment or representation of abstract ideas or ideals in the form of a story or picture.

33. B: False

   You know that Madeira's a province of Portugal, so Madeira's a Portuguese wine.

34. C: Can't tell

    This answer happens to be true – the wine is *maderised* (oxidised through heating) during the *estufagem* process that follows fermentation – but you can't deduce this from the passage.

35. C: Can't tell

    The passage discusses the impact of phylloxera only on Madeira, not on the wine industry in general.

    In fact, phylloxera did have a devastating effect across the entire Old World wine industry, and only grafting onto resistant rootstocks allowed the trade to survive to the present day.

36. A: True

    The passage says as much.

37. A: True

    You know that China adopted a policy of letting some people get rich before others.

    This concept is a primitive form of capitalism – although in reality China's central government continues to exert major control over the economic experiment.

38. C: Can't tell

    The passage suggests that this is the case in China, but you can't generalise from this specific case. The precise effects of how capital and income distribute across different groups under different economic scenarios remain a complex area of debate among economists.

39. C: Can't tell

    The passage specifically describes PPP as being only one view, and so you can't make absolute statements about the utility of PPP. However, intuitively this answer makes sense.

40. A: True

    You know that despite significant income inequality, price levels in the poor areas are much lower than in the rich areas, which mitigates the effect in terms of PPP. Inflation would cause prices to rise, which, given the lower level of income in the poor areas, would impact on poor people the most.

    In fact, China's government is highly aware of this risk (partly because it fears loss of government authority in poor areas) and tries to manipulate the market to dampen the effect of inflation in these areas.

41. A: Aristotle

    The sentence is: 'Near the end of his life, Alexander the Great ordered the execution as a traitor of Aristotle's grandnephew Callisthenes and this and other things soured the relationship between the king and his master.' In other words, Alexander had Aristotle's nephew killed, which soured his relationship with Aristotle.

42. C: Aristotle thought he'd be safe on Euboea.

    Aristotle escaped to Euboea saying that he wouldn't suffer the same fate as Socrates, meaning that he thought he'd be safe on Euboea. The text says that the execution of Callisthenes soured the relationship between Alexander and Aristotle, suggested that their relationship had once been warm (A). It's not stated what Alexander died from, merely that he died in Babylon in 323 BC (B). When Aristotle fled Athens, he cited Socrates, but that need not mean that he had met with Socrates (D).

43. D: After Alexander's death, Aristotle feared for his life.

    The text says that, after Alexander's death, Aristotle was denounced for not holding the gods in honour. He then fled Athens, saying that he didn't want to suffer the same fate as Socrates, who was tried and executed. The Lyceum can't be another name for the peripatetic school (A), since Theophrastus was already leader of the peripatetic school when Aristotle designated him as head of the Lyceum. The text does say that Alexander ordered the execution of Aristotle's nephew, but from this it can't be inferred that Alexander disliked Aristotle (B). The text only says that Euboea was the homeland of Aristotle's mother's family. This doesn't necessarily mean that Aristotle was born on Euboea (C).

44. A: Aristotle disliked Theophrastus.

    Aristotle wouldn't have made Theophrastus the chief beneficiary of his will if he'd disliked him. The text says that, 'after Alexander's death in Babylon in 323BC, anti-Macedonian feelings in Athens flared up, and Eurydemon the hierophant denounced Aristotle for not holding the gods in honour', suggesting that Eurydemon had anti-Macedonian feelings (B). Eurydemon's accusations would probably not have prompted Aristotle to flee Athens if most people living in those times hadn't been religious (C). Aristotle was a philosopher, since, upon fleeing, he explained that he would 'not allow the Athenians to sin twice against philosophy' (D).

Quantitative Reasoning

1. D: 70.8%

   Seven MPs claimed between £125k and £149k. A further seven MPs claimed between £150k and £174k. A final three MPs claimed above £175k. Therefore, 7 + 7 + 3 = 17 out of a total of 24 MPs who claimed at least £125k. As a percentage, 17 ÷ 24 × 100 = 70.8% to one decimal place.

2. B: 5:7

   A total of 7 + 3 = 10 MPs claimed £150k or more, which means that 24 – 10 = 14 MPs claimed less than £150k. The ratio is 10:14, which you can simplify to 5:7.

3. D: £119k

   This category contains only three MPs. If the total of their three claims is £340k and the largest claim is £121k, the sum of the other two is (340k – 121k) = 219k.

   The question asks what is the maximum that one of these two MPs could have claimed. You need to assume that the other MP claims the minimum to remain in the category – 100k. The maximum remaining is therefore 219k – 100k = £119k.

4. D: £79 million

   The old total was £98 million and has reduced by 19%. The new total is therefore [98 million × (100 – 19)] ÷ 100 = £79 million.

5. D: 133

   This question is a test of your ability to calculate an arithmetic mean:

   (68 + 235 + 194 + 217 + 53 + 46 + 117) ÷ 7 = 133 in thousands and to the nearest whole thousand

6. C: April

   You can calculate this answer by adding together the monthly data until you go beyond the 600,000th job. You pass this total in April.

7. B: 1:1.9

   Jobs added in June and July: 46 + 117 = 163

   Jobs added in January and February: 68 + 235 = 303

   The ratio is 163:303, which you can simplify to 1:1.9 approximately.

8. C: 130

The second quarter is April, May and June. The average gain in these months is $(217 + 53 + 46) \div 3 = 105.3$ thousand to one decimal place. A 23 per cent increase on this average is $105.3 \times 123 \div 100 = 130$ thousand (approximately).

9. C: One too many in the >15% band

You can derive this answer by doing the work that the hypothetical analyst should have done and drawing up the table correctly.

10. C: 7%

The average is $(5.2 + 8.6 + 8.5 + 7.5 + 5.6 + 6.5) \div 6 = 7\%$ (approximately).

11. E: 2,250%

This question is more difficult than it appears. The question contains lots of different percentage figures, which can be confusing. Japan's figure is 0.2 per cent and South Korea's figure is 4.7 per cent. Japan's inflation rate has to be $(4.7 - 0.2) = 4.5$ percentage points higher to match South Korea – but the question doesn't ask you to calculate this. The question asks you by what percentage Japan's inflation rate has to increase to in order to match South Korea's $4.5 \div 0.2 \times 100 = 2,250\%$.

12. A: 7%

India's inflation is 8.6 per cent but contributes a relative weighting of only $1.4 \div (1.4 + 5)$. China's inflation is 6.5 per cent but contributes $5 \div (1.4 + 5)$. The total combined rate of inflation is therefore:

$(8.6 \times 1.4 \div 6.4) + (6.5 \times 5 \div 6.4) = 7\%$ (approximately)

13. D: 285

The mode is the score that appears most frequently, which is 285.

14. E: 283

You calculate this answer by summing all the scores and dividing by the sample size: $5,662 \div 20 = 283$, to the nearest whole stroke.

15. C: 65%

In all, 13 scores are less than 286, so the percentage is $13 \div 20 \times 100 = 65\%$.

16. B: 31%

Odds of 5:11 mean that for every 5 times KB wins, JD wins 11 times. In other words, out of a total of 16 games, KB wins 5 games. As a percentage, this chance of winning is $5 \div 16 \times 100 = 31\%$ to the nearest whole per cent.

17. C: 35

    12 furlongs = 12 ÷ 8 = 1.5 miles

    2 minutes and 35 seconds = 155 seconds = (155 ÷ 3,600) hours

    The calculation for speed is distance ÷ time = 1.5 ÷ (155 ÷ 3,600) = 35 miles per hour (approximately).

18. B: 155.3 seconds

    This question is quite challenging. Pour Moi completes the course of 12 furlongs in 2 minutes and 35 seconds.

    12 furlongs = 12 ÷ 8 × 1,760 = 2,640 yards

    Therefore, Carlton House covers 2,640 – 5 = 2,635 yards in those same 155 seconds. You can then calculate the average speed of Carlton House and use the total race distance to calculate the horse's time to complete the course.

    You can also take a mathematical shortcut. Because the horse's speed is constant throughout the race, you can scale up the time that the winning horse took, based on the relative distances of the winner and the third-placed horse:

    2,640 ÷ 2,635 × 155 = 155.3 seconds

19. D: 68 yards

    If Workforce won in 2 minutes 31 seconds (= 151 seconds), you need to know how far Pour Moi travelled in that time to find out the distance by which Workforce beat Pour Moi.

    You know that each horse's speed is uniform, so you need to do a simple calculation based on the ratio of the two horses' individual winning times and the total course distance:

    151 ÷ 155 × 2,640 (course length) = 2,572 yards

    The difference between this and the course length gives you the hypothetical winning margin:

    2,640 – 2,572 = 68 yards

20. E: 3 minutes 9 seconds

    The St Leger course distance is 1 mile, 6 furlongs and 132 yards, or:

    1,760 + (6 ÷ 8 × 1,760) + 132 = 1,760 + 1,320 + 132 = 3,212 yards

    Pour Moi covered 2,640 yards in 155 seconds to win the Derby. The time that the horse takes to cover 3,212 yards at the same speed is:

    3,212 ÷ (2,640 ÷ 155) = 3,212 ÷ 2,640 × 155 = 189 seconds = 3 minutes 9 seconds

21. B: 9:5

    In 1997, Blue Skies took 15.7 per cent of the market, and Big Green took 8.5 per cent. The ratio between the two is 15.7:8.5, or approximately 1.8:1, which is equivalent to 9:5.

22. D: The combined market share of the three supermarkets suffered a fall in 2009.

    A, B and C are demonstrably false, and E cannot be proved from the information in the chart.

23. D: £21.6 billion

    125 billion × 17.3% = £21.6 billion

24. A: 6.7%

    In 1997, the greatest market share was that of Blue Skies at 15.2 per cent, and the lowest market share was that of Big Green at 8.5 per cent. The range is therefore 15.2 − 8.5 = 6.7%.

25. B: £0.81

    12 kWh per day is 12 × 30 = 360 kWh usage per month.

    With quarterly billing, Catherine pays (360 × 3.81p) + (30 × 29.97p) = 2,270.7p = £22.71 to the nearest penny.

    With monthly direct debit, Catherine pays (360 × 3.59p) + (30 × 29.92p) = 2,190p = £21.90 to the nearest penny.

    The difference is 22.71 − 21.90 = £0.81.

26. E: £52.24

    Off-peak daily use is (12 × 1 ÷ 3) = 4 kWh. Peak daily use is 12 − 4 = 8 kWh.

    Monthly cost of off-peak use = 30 × 4 × 7.12p = 854.4p

    Monthly cost of peak use = 30 × 8 × 15.01p = 3,602.4p

    Monthly standing charge = 30 × 25.56p = 766.8p

    The total cost is 854.4 + 3,602.4 + 766.8 = 5,223.6p = £52.24 to the nearest penny.

27. C: £37.26

    New daily consumption is (12 × 80) ÷ 100 = 9.6.

    Off-peak daily use is 9.6 × 60% = 5.76 kWh.

    Peak daily use is 9.6 − 5.76 = 3.84 kWh.

    Monthly cost of off-peak use = 30 × 5.76 × 7.12p = 1,230.3p

    Monthly cost of peak use = 30 × 3.84 × 15.01p = 1,729.1p to one decimal place

    Monthly standing charge cost = 30 × 25.56p = 766.8p

    The total cost is 1,230.3 + 1,729.1 + 766.8 = 3,726.2p = £37.26 to the nearest penny.

28. C: If Catherine uses 200 kWh per month, Isis Energy can undercut Midlands Energy's price.

    You can prove that all the other options are true. More straightforwardly, from the calculations required for the previous questions, you can see that Isis can't possibly be cheaper than Midlands at Catherine's level of consumption.

29. D: 7

    The range is the difference between the maximum and minimum values: 82.7 − 75.7 = 7 years.

30. E: 81.5

    The assumption regarding equal regional weighting lets you simply calculate the arithmetic mean to find the answer. In real life, the different regions contribute different numbers of people to the overall total, so you'd have to weight their contribution to the overall English average by those populations. Your task in this question is much simpler:

    (80.1 + 80.3 + 81.0 + 81.3 + 81.1 + 82.3 + 82.0 + 82.4 + 82.7) ÷ 9 = 81.5 to one decimal place

31. C: 5.9%

    (82.0 − 77.4) ÷ 77.4 × 100 = 5.9% to one decimal place

32. B: A man born in the South West will, on average, live a longer life than one born in the North East.

    It's nice when the correct option is early on in the list and you can stop checking the other propositions! However, if you do work through all the options to double-check, you can see that all the other statements are false.

33. D: 576

    The long wall measures 5 m × 2 m. Because each module measures 1.2 m × 0.85, you can fit a total of eight modules against the wall.

    Trying to calculate this answer by working out the area of the wall and dividing by the area of the module is a mistake, because the modules by definition are the smallest component of the rack and so you can't break them up. Instead, you need to calculate how many modules fit lengthwise (5 ÷ 1.2 = 4.17 = 4 rounded down) and how many modules fit height-wise (2 ÷ 0.85 = 2.35 = 2 rounded down) and multiply the two figures: 4 × 2 = 8.

    Each module contains 72 bottles, so the total storage space is 72 × 8 = 576.

34. C: £1,152

    You already know that George needs eight racks, so the total cost excluding VAT is 8 × 120 = £960. Adding in the VAT at 20 per cent gives 960 × 120 ÷ 100 = £1,152.

35. B: £385

The cost to purchase and install is £550. Amortised over ten years, this is $550 \div 10 = £55$ per year.

The cost of electricity per year is $6,600 \times 5p = 3,3000p = £330$.

Adding the two costs together gives $330 + 55 = £385$.

36. D: £28,512

Three cases of Alsatian Gewürztraminer at £26 per bottle cost $(3 \times 12) \times 26 = £936$.

Two cases of Hermitage at £720 per case cost $2 \times 720 = £1,440$.

One case of fine Bordeaux at £99 per bottle costs $(1 \times 12) \times 99 = £1,188$.

The total cost is $936 + 1,440 + 1,188 = £3,564$.

The average cost per bottle is $3,564 \div (6 \times 12) = £49.50$.

You know that George's cellar contains 576 bottles, so the total cost to fill the cellar, based on the average cost, is $£49.50 \times 576 = £28,512$.

Abstract Reasoning

1, A

Explanation
The number of circles decreases by one each time, while the number of crosses increases by one.

2, B

Explanation
The centre always stays the same. In the first instance, the arms rotate by 90 degrees clockwise. In the second instance, they rotate a further 180 degrees either clockwise or anticlockwise. In the third instance, they rotate a further 90 degrees clockwise, placing them into the same position as in square 1. You can assume that they will next rotate by 90 degrees clockwise – an assumption confirmed by the available answer options.

3, B; **4,** A

Explanation
In Set A, the top half of the square is reflected in the bottom half. In Set B, the left half of the square is reflected in the right half. Note that it's not a true reflection: the shapes reflected from top to bottom aren't inverted. That might have made it too easy!

5, D

Explanation
Each time, the central circle shifts from black to white and white to black, and the peripheral shapes rotate anticlockwise by one position.

6, neither set; **7,** Set B; **8,** Set B; **9,** Set A; **10,** neither set

Explanation
All the objects in Set A have outer edges with interruptions. All the objects in Set B have solid outer edges. The exact nature of the overall shape, the colour and the orientation show no consistent features of commonality.

Test shapes 7 and 8 have only objects with solid uninterrupted outer edges and so fall within Set B. Test shape 9 has only interrupted outlines and so falls into Set A. Test shapes 6 and 10 contain objects with both solid and interrupted outlines and so fall into neither set.

11, neither set; **12**, neither set; **13**, neither set; **14**, Set B; **15**, Set A

Explanation

All the objects in set A have three edges. All the objects in Set B have four edges. Test shape 15 contains only three-edged objects and so is in Set A. Test shape 14 has only four-edged objects and so is in Set B. Test shapes 11, 12 and 13 contain objects with varying numbers of edges and so fall into neither set.

16, neither set; **17**, neither set; **18**, Set B; **19**, neither set; **20**, Set A

Explanation

All the examples in Set A contain a shape that's internally replicated in the same colour. Any extra shapes on the outside have the opposite colour from the main shape. For instance, the top-left item contains a large white circle with a smaller white inner circle and a black outer shape (in this case, also a circle).

All the examples in Set B contain a shape that's internally replicated in the opposite colour. The extra shape on the outside has the same colour as the main shape. For instance, the top-left item contains a large white hexagon with a smaller black inner hexagon and no second outer object. The top-right item contains a large white triangle with a smaller black inner triangle and a white outer shape (in this case, a triangle).

The placement and orientation of the large object within the box are irrelevant. Any other shapes in each item show no consistent features of commonality.

Test shape 20 contains a large white object that's replicated internally by a smaller white item and a second outer object in the opposite colour from the big shape, and so is in Set A. Test shape 18 has a large object that's internally replicated with a smaller black object and a second outer object in the same colour as the big shape, and so it fits in Set B.

Test shape 16 has a smaller object that isn't an exact internal replication, and so belongs to neither set. Test shapes 17 and 19 have no internal replication at all and so belong to neither set.

21, C

Explanation

The superimposed shapes shift in order. The innermost shape becomes the middle shape, the middle shape becomes the outermost shape, and the outermost shape becomes the innermost shape. In addition, the new innermost shape adopts the colour or marking of the old outermost square, and vice versa.

22, B

Explanation

The superimposed shapes shift in order. The innermost shape is interchanged with the outermost shape, and the second shape is interchanged with the third shape. The colours and shadings are red herrings.

23, A

Explanation

Each basic shape gains one side.

24, D

Explanation

Each shape gains a segment.

25, D

Explanation

The square moves down by one quarter of the length of the line each time. In contrast, the circle moves up by one quarter of the length of the line each time.

26, Set A; **27**, neither set; **28**, Set B; **29**, Set B; **30**, neither set

Explanation

All the examples in set A contain only items with right-angles. All the examples in Set B contain only items with no right-angles. The exact nature of the overall shape, the colour and the orientation show no consistent features of commonality.

Test shape 26 contains only objects with right-angles and so belongs to Set A. Test shapes 28 and 29 have no right-angled figures and so belong to Set B. Test shapes 27 and 30 include both objects with and objects without right-angles and so don't fit into either set.

31, Set A; **32**, Set B; **33**, Set A; **34**, Set B; **35**, Set B

Explanation

In Set A, if you can see a circle, you also see an arrow. Conversely, if you see no circle, you don't see an arrow. Set B's rules are the opposite: if you can see a circle, you don't see an arrow; but if you see no circle, you can see an arrow. The colour and the direction of the arrow are irrelevant.

Test shapes 31 and 33 contain both circles and arrows and so are in Set A. Test shapes 32 and 35 contain no circle but do have arrows, and so are in Set B. Test shape 34 has a circle but no arrow and so is in Set B.

36, B

Explanation

Each shape moves down a line, with the shape on the bottom line moving back to the top line. With each movement, the triangle oscillates from left to right, the circle from centre to left, and the square from right to left.

37, A

Explanation

Each time, the square moves one line to the right and oscillates from top to bottom; the circle moves *two* lines to the right, and oscillates from bottom to top.

38, C

Explanation

Each time, the three crosses rotate by 90 degrees clockwise. The lines are a red herring.

39, B

Explanation

Each shape gains one side *and* adds a segment.

40, B

Explanation

The figure rotates by 90 degrees clockwise. The shaded central circle becomes a white square, the peripheral white square becomes shaded, and the peripheral black circle contained in the square (which itself doesn't change colour) becomes white.

41, neither set; **42**, Set B; **43**, Set A; **44**, Set A; **45**, neither set

Explanation

The pictures in Set A all contain one fewer objects than the the number of edges of the object with the most edges. The pictures in Set B all have the same number of objects as the object with most edges.

Test shapes 43 and 44 fall into Set A. Test shape 42 is in Set B. Test shapes 41 and 45 obey neither set's rules.

46, C

Explanation

The shapes rotate by 180 degrees in position. The circles become triangles, and the triangle becomes a square – in other words, each shape gains at least one side.

47, B; **48**, B

Explanation

In Set A, the smaller angle between the hour hand and the minute hand of the clock is always greater than 90 degrees. In Set B, it's always 90 degrees or less.

49, A

Explanation

The white triangles become black squares, and the black circles become white circles (and it's fair to assume that the opposite applies). The relative positions of the shapes are a red herring.

50, C

Explanation

Angular shapes are swapped for non-angular shapes and vice versa.

51, Set A; **52**, Set B; **53**, neither set; **54**, Set B; **55**, neither set

Explanation

If the identical objects are in vertical or horizontal alignment, the shape falls into Set A. If the identical objects are in diagonal alignment, the shape is in Set B.

Test shape 51 is in Set A. Test shapes 52 and 54 are in Set B. Test shapes 53 and 55 have no identical shapes and so belong to neither set.

Decision Analysis

1. B: Pass the ball to the striker.

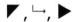

= Ball, Pass, Striker

= Ball pass to striker

= Pass the ball to the striker

2. C: Pass to midfield then to the striker then shoot.

↳↓ △↓↳, ▶, ⟨

= Pass, Midfielder, Pass, Striker, Shoot

= Pass to midfield, pass to the striker, shoot

= Pass to midfield then to the striker then shoot

3. E: Keep possession.

⇉(▲, ↳, ▼, ▲)

= Increase (Cannons, Pass, Ball, Cannons)

= Do more of (cannons passing the ball to each other)

= Keep possession

4. D: The referee's an idiot.

⇉ ⌃, ↻

= Increase Disapprove, Referee

= Greatly disapprove of referee

= The referee's an idiot

This translation takes some liberties with the literal decoded translation, forcing you to equate a general sense of great disapproval with considering the referee to be stupid, but the answer is the best fit of the options available and conveys the gist of the message.

None of the other options fits the code. Nothing suggests 'soon', as mentioned in option A. Options B and C are too specific for the code, mentioning the opposition or the manager's players. Option E discusses bribery, a concept not conveyed by the code.

5. A: Send off that opposition player, referee!

🖎, ‿, ⇉(⌢ ⇆), ▼

= Referee, Whistle, Increase (Disapprove Talk), Opponent

= Referee, blow whistle and severely tell off opposing player

= Referee should blow whistle and send off opposition player

= Send off that opposition player, referee!

You need to translate the code into a casual vernacular phrase. Sending off a player's not the same as severely telling off the player, but the two phrases share something of the same meaning. None of the other options remotely fits the code. You don't need to know the rules of football or even know what sending off means to decode this message, because you can eliminate the other options as unsatisfactory translations.

6. E: I want two defenders to stay near the goalposts to defend this corner.

◀◀(⌣), ←↖

= Defender Defender (Goalposts), Defend Corner

= Two defenders at goalposts, defend corner

= I want two defenders to stay near the goalposts to defend this corner

7. C: Midfield needs to attack faster.

(△ △), →↻

= (Midfielder Midfield), Attack Fast

= Midfielders plural, attack fast

= Midfield needs to attack faster

8. A: We need to score one more than the opposition does.

(▲ ⇧)⇉, ▼ ⇧

= (Cannons Score) Increase, Opponent Score

= Our score needs to be more than the opposition's score

= We need to score one more than the opposition does

9. B: Referee, the opposing defender handballed!

↻, ▼◀, ⊢▶

= Referee, Opponent Defender, Hand Ball

= Referee, the opposing defender handballed!

Option A lacks the specificity of mentioning the defender. Option C adds in more elaboration than necessary compared with option B. Options D and E contain elements of distracting the referee, which aren't included in the code.

10. C: Tell that idiot striker to just hit the ball into the net!

⚡▶, ∧, (⌒⇉)▶

= Shoot ball, Net, (Disapprove Increase) Striker

= Shoot the ball into the net, (I disapprove greatly) striker

= Tell that idiot striker to just hit the ball into the net!

11. E: The keeper saves from the striker, but the midfielder scores on the rebound.

▶⚡, ▽←, △⇗

= Striker Shoot, Goalkeeper Defend, Midfielder Score

= The striker shoots, the goalkeeper defends, the midfielder scores

= The keeper saved from the striker, but the midfielder scored on the rebound

Options C and D convey something of the same message, but option D omits elements of the code and option C gets the order of events wrong.

12. A: ⇆, (⇆↔)▶, ◀

= Talk, (Talk Walk) Striker, Defender

= Tell me, (tell walk) striker, defender

= Tell me if I need to tell the striker to walk, for a defender

= Tell me if you want me to substitute a striker for a defender

Option C is superficially similar but lacks the crucial element of asking the person receiving the message to talk to the manager about whether the manager should request the substitution.

13. D: Run into the opposition's half.

$$\circlearrowleft \leftrightarrow, \; \blacktriangledown \ddagger$$

 = Fast Walk, Opponent Halfway Line

 = Run, opposition's side of the halfway line

 = Run into the opposition's half

14. C: Score two goals in this half.

$$(\; \hat{\mathbb{m}} \; \hat{\mathbb{m}} \;)(\; \underset{\smile}{} \; \ddagger \;)$$

 = (Score Score) (Whistle Halfway Line)

 = Score twice (whistle halfway line)

 = Score twice when the whistle is halfway

 = Score twice in this half

The need to transpose a pitch object (the halfway line) into a time (this half) underlines how ambiguity can creep into decoding from a symbolic cipher, but this answer is the best (or least worst) option from the list.

Option A has the essential element of scoring twice, but specifies that this should happen in each half. The code, even stretched to its limit, only talks about one half. Option B has two goals in total but spreads them across the two halves, whereas their grouping together in the code is best interpreted as scoring closer together. Option D discusses winning, which isn't in the code. Option E mentions a rematch, which isn't hinted at by the code.

15. A: $\blacktriangledown \nwarrow, \; \circlearrowleft \underset{\smile}{}, \; \hat{\mathbb{m}}$

 = Ball Corner, Referee Whistle, Score

 = Ball on corner spot, referee blows his whistle, then score

 = Place the ball on the corner spot and score when the referee blows his whistle

16. B: Midfield needs to pass up to the striker so he can head a goal.

$$(\triangle \triangle) \vdash, \; \blacktriangleright, \; \rightarrow | \; \hat{\mathbb{m}}$$

 = (Midfielder Midfielder) Pass, Striker, Head Score

 = Midfielders pass to striker, head a goal

 = Midfield needs to pass up to the striker so he can head a goal

17. D: I need everyone to run faster, pass more and get the ball to the strikers.

▲ (⇉ ((↔ ○), ↪)), ▶ ▶

= Cannons (Increase ((Walk Fast), Pass)), Striker Striker

= Cannons (increase (run, pass)), strikers

= Cannons (run faster, pass more), strikers

= I need everyone to run faster, pass more, and get the ball to strikers

In this case, the manager omits the code for ball, because he implies the meaning in his request for passing. The manager may have used the code for 'fast' to encourage his players to run faster; by using the code for 'increase' instead, he can apply the term to both 'run' and 'pass', gaining in concision.

18. E: Well done, lads; now attack, attack, attack!

↘ ▲ , ⇉ →

= Approve Cannons, Increase Attack

= Well done, lads; now attack, attack, attack!

19. B: The referee will blow his whistle any minute now; hang on!

○ ⇉ (↘ ‿), ⇉ ←

= Fast Increase (Referee Whistle), Increase Defend

= Imminent (referee will blow whistle), more defending

= The referee will blow his whistle any minute now, defend more until then

= The referee will blow his whistle any minute now; hang on!

20. A: We need our defence to slow the game down.

▲ (◀ ◀), ○ ⇉

= Cannons (Defender Defender), Slow Increase

= Our defence, more slow

= We need our defence to slow the game down

21. C: Get our midfield to send more penetrating crosses to the strikers.

$$\leftrightarrows, \quad \blacktriangle(\,\triangle\,\triangle\,), \rightarrow(\vdash\!\!\vdash), \blacktriangle(\blacktriangleright\blacktriangleright\,)$$

= Talk, Cannons (Midfielder Midfielder), Attack (Pass Pass), Cannons (Striker Striker)

= Talk, our midfield, attacking passes, our strikers

= Get our midfield to send more penetrating crosses to the strikers

22. E: The opponents managed to get the referee to send our defender off the pitch.

$$\blacktriangledown\blacktriangledown, \leftrightarrows, \circlearrowleft, (\,\smile^{\frown})\leftrightarrow, \blacktriangleleft$$

= Opponent Opponent, Talk, Referee, (Whistle Disapprove)Walk, Defender

= The opponents, talk, referee to blow his whistle in disapproval to walk defender

= The opponents talked to the referee to get him to send off our defender

= The opponents managed to get the referee to send our defender off the pitch

Option D conveys a similar meaning, but the code includes the symbol for referee, so the optimal translation should explicitly include that if possible. Option E is therefore a closer translation, making it the correct answer.

23. C: Owner

and

D: Sell

You can't possibly convey these two terms using the current code. You can convey the term 'play' by combining all the elements of a game (attack, defend, score, pass). You can convey 'better' by using 'approve' and 'increase'. You can convey 'lot of you' simply by using the code for 'cannons'. Conveying property rights isn't possible with the limited code.

24. A: Match

    and

    D: Calm

    This cliché-ridden bit of manager-speak requires you to translate the essential meaning of the idioms rather than translate them literally. 'Over the moon' requires you to convey a sense of extreme happiness, which you can do through judicious use of the terms for 'approve' and possibly 'talk'. You can convey 'giving 110 per cent', or trying one's hardest, using the terms for 'attack', 'defend' and 'increase' – and possibly 'approve' too.

    Conveying a sense of taking each match as it comes is much harder. You need to translate a calm and methodical approach to each game. 'Calm' is therefore a useful term to have. The term 'match' is also helpful. Although you can just about use a similar technique to the one we describe in answer 23 to group all the elements of a match to translate the concept, doing so is more convoluted than the solution for the other potential answers in the list (calm excepted).

25. A: Get one of our defenders to cover the goalpost nearest the corner, and another to stand next to the keeper and block the net.

    ▲ ◀(↖ ⊐), (▲ ◀ ▽)←⌃

    = Cannons Defender(Corner Goalpost), (Cannons Defender Keeper) Defend Net

    = One of our defenders (Corner Goalpost), (another of our defenders and our keeper) defend the net

    = Get one of our defenders to cover the goalpost nearest the corner, and another to stand next to the keeper and block the net

26. C: It's the last minute of the match, we have a corner . . . and score!

    ◡ ⇉(↺ ‿), ▲ ↖, ⇪

    = Fast Increase (Referee Whistle), Cannons Corner, Score

    = The referee's about to blow his whistle, we have a corner, score

    = It's the last minute of the match, we have a corner . . . and score!

27. C: Pass to the striker to shoot with his head.

= Pass, Striker, Shoot Head

= Pass to the striker to shoot with his head

28. A: The striker doesn't want to shoot the penalty.

$\nleftarrow, \uparrow, \blacktriangleright, \overline{\wedge}$

= Shoot, Penalty Spot, Striker, Disapprove.

'Penalty spot' becomes simply 'penalty', and 'disapprove' can be used to say 'does not want'.

= Shoot the penalty the striker doesn't want

= The striker doesn't want to shoot the penalty

Situational Judgement Test

1, D; **2**, A; **3**, A; **4**, C; **5**, A; **6**, A

Discussion:

In some cases, it's appropriate for doctors to encourage patients to consent to disclosures that are necessary for their own protection (answer 2). Dr Osode should also do his best to provide Mrs Patel with the information and support she needs to help her deal with or resolve the situation (answer 3).

On the other hand, a competent adult has the right to refuse to consent to disclosure, even if that decision leaves that person at risk of serious harm (answer 4).

Disclosure without consent may be justified if others are at risk. Dr Patel should therefore establish whether Mrs Patel has any children or vulnerable adults living with her (answer 5). This is the very least that he'd be expected to do (answer 1).

In addition, doctors must keep clear and accurate records, reporting the information exchanged with patients as well as any relevant findings (answer 6).

7, D; **8**, D; **9**, A; **10**, D

Discussion:

Doctors shouldn't accept any gift or hospitality that may affect or be seen to affect the way they care for their patients (answer 7). Furthermore, doctors mustn't pursue personal relationships with former patients who were vulnerable at the time of the professional relationship (answers 7, 8 and 10). Mrs Patel is still in counselling and likely to be very vulnerable.

The only appropriate course of action is to politely decline her invitation (answer 9).

11, A; **12**, A; **13**, C; **14**, A

Discussion:

The main reception of the hospital is a very inappropriate place in which to break bad news to a patient's relative. Before anything, Marisa ought to consider Emma's comfort and privacy, for example by finding a consultation room in which to hold their meeting (answer 11).

Before breaking the bad news, Marisa ought to find out how much Emma already knows about her father's condition. This will help her to frame their conversation and avoid causing Emma undue upset (answer 12).

In breaking the bad news, Marisa ought to be as accurate, sensitive and sympathetic as possible, regardless of whether Emma feels close to her father. However, Emma's closeness to her father isn't totally irrelevant: for example, if Emma feels very close to her father, she may benefit from a course of counselling (answer 13).

In such a situation, it's easy to overlook Mr Glover's right to confidentiality. However unlikely, it's possible that Mr Glover actually objects to his daughter being told the details of his condition (answer 14).

15, A; **16**, C; **17**, A; **18**, B

Discussion:

The central issue is whether, in this situation, Mr Firkin has the capacity to make decisions about his care. If he does, then his decisions should be respected, regardless of his daughter's (or indeed the doctor's) opinion (answer 15). The fact that Mr Firkin has recently been diagnosed with dementia is of minor importance, since it doesn't preclude him from having the capacity to decide about his care (answer 16).

If Mr Firkin is suffering from a potentially life-threatening condition, then his need to go to hospital is much greater, and the degree of capacity that he requires to make that decision much higher (answer 17). Close carers or close relatives are best placed to know the exact severity and impact of a patient's symptoms and also what the patient himself would have wanted had he not lacked the capacity to decide about his care.

Although Amanda's concern isn't the central issue, it's an important factor to take into account (answer 18).

19, B; **20**, A; **21**, D; **22**, C

Discussion:

In the first instance, the group should seek to resolve the issue by raising it with Liz. To do this in private is more sensitive (answers 19 and 20).

Regardless of whether the project is advancing well, Liz's failure to pull her weight is impacting on the other students in the group. Moreover, Liz may have issues that need to be addressed, either personal issues or issues with working as a team (answer 21).

To discuss the issue with the course leader without having first sought to resolve or even discuss it with Liz would be very premature (answer 22).

23, D; **24**, A; **25**, D; **26**, D

Discussion:

The best response is to reassure and pacify the child, and his own mother is in the best position to do this (answer 24). To carry on with the examination anyway would be counterproductive, because it would further distress the child and make him even less cooperative (answer 23).

To give up on the examination and rely on the history alone could potentially have serious, even fatal, consequences (answer 25). To attend to other patients and return in a couple of hours could have similarly serious consequences (answer 26).

27, D; **28**, D; **29**, A; **30**, A

Discussion:

Linda's already caused the patient significant pain and distress. Instead of trying one or several more times to insert the cannula, she should seek help from a more experienced colleague who can minimise the patient's suffering (answer 30). The clinical need for a cannula is critical: if the need is great then Linda should seek help as soon as possible (answer 29).

Linda's concerns for her image or reputation shouldn't affect her clinical decision making (answer 27).

As a junior foundation year 1 (FY1) doctor, Linda clearly needs more practice inserting cannulas, but, again, this shouldn't impact on her clinical decision making (answer 28).

31, D; **32**, D; **33**, D; **34** A

Discussion:

To tell Mr Jones (who's in pain and has been waiting for almost six hours) that his behaviour is inappropriate and selfish is insensitive and only likely to make matters worse (answer 31). To promise that he'll be seen next is unfair to other patients. Moreover, Angelina isn't in a position to make or honour that promise (answer 32).

The appropriate course of action is to provide Mr Jones with an explanation and an apology in a bid to quell or contain his anger (answer 34). However, in so doing, it would be very unprofessional to start scoring political points or blaming managerial colleagues (answer 33).

35, C; **36**, D; **37**, B; **38**, A;

Discussion:

Luke's behaviour is not only unsympathetic and uncaring, but also offensive and unacceptable – especially for a future medical practitioner. Therefore, to do nothing at all would be very inappropriate (answer 36). To subtly change the subject may improve matters a little, but without really addressing the problem (answer 35).

Laura ought to tell Luke to stop making such jokes. To do this, she would be better off taking Luke aside so as to minimise his embarrassment and preserve friendly relations with him (answers 37 and 38).

39, C; **40**, C; **41**, D; **42**, A

Discussion:

Jess has taken an overdose and is therefore at risk of killing herself. As a very junior (FY1) doctor, David isn't in a position to assess Jess's degree of risk or authorise her discharge. He ought therefore to call for a senior or specialist opinion (answer 42).

Jess's risk factors, for example her mental state and the type and size of her overdose, don't invalidate David seeking an opinion from a more experienced doctor, although they may have some bearing on its urgency (answers 39 and 40).

Jess's apparent cheerfulness isn't to be taken at face value, because it could be a mask aimed at deceiving David into discharging her (answer 41).

43, D; **44**, C; **45**, B; **46**, A; **47**, C

Discussion:

The head nurse's behaviour is highly inappropriate and very likely to adversely affect Samantha's professional relationships with the nursing staff and, by extension, patient care. To say nothing would therefore be very inappropriate (answer 43).

Samantha ought to raise the issue with the head nurse. To do so there and then, while not strictly inappropriate, would risk antagonising the head nurse and making matters worse (answer 45). Ideally, Samantha ought to have a quiet word with the nurse in an office or side room (answer 46).

To report the head nurse to the hospital authorities without first having tried to resolve the situation would be an overreaction (answer 44).

To invite some of the nurses out for a drink might indeed make her more popular, but wouldn't address the head nurse's bad behavior (answer 47).

48, D; **49**, D; **50**, A; **51**, C

Discussion:

Although Andrew is disappointed with Mr Kumar, Mr Kumar may have had good reasons for providing the patient with the sort of explanation that he did. Alternatively, Mr Kumar's explanation may have sufficed in the context of a clinical consultation. The best course of action is for Andrew to wait until the consultation is finished and discuss the issue with Mr Kumar. This could be a good learning opportunity for Andrew (answer 50).

To wait until the consultation has finished and then provide the patient with a 'better' explanation would be very inappropriate and potentially undermine the patient's trust in his surgeon (answer 48). To interrupt the consultation for the same purpose would be just as inappropriate, if not more so (answer 49).

For Andrew to ask the medical school to attach him to another consultant on the basis of this situation would be a gross overreaction that may offend Mr Kumar (answer 51).

52, D; **53**, A; **54**, A; **55**, D

Discussion:

Doctors may disclose information to a known sexual contact of a patient with HIV if that contact is at risk of infection. However, they should weigh the benefits and harms of disclosing confidential information without consent.

In this case, Dr Stewart ought to talk to Mr Brown before he considers making a disclosure of this type to Mr Poole. Dr Stewart should first try to persuade Mr Brown to tell Mr Poole himself (answers 52, 53 and 55).

In addition, he should also advise Mr Poole to have protected sex (answer 54).

56, D; **57**, B; **58**, D; **59**, A

Discussion:

Although Nancy's vulnerable and at risk, she still has capacity. Dr Sullivan should abide by Nancy's decision not to disclose, even if it places Nancy (but nobody else) at risk of serious harm (answer 57 and 58).

However, Dr Sullivan ought to encourage Nancy to consent to disclosure and do his best to support Nancy to make a decision in her own best interests, for example by arranging contact with support agencies (answer 59).

All patients are entitled to care and treatment to meet their clinical needs, and doctors shouldn't withhold treatment from patients who need it, whatever the circumstances (answer 56).

60, A; **61**, A; **62**, D; **63**, A

Discussion:

Dr Tzakanikis must ensure that the referral is what Mr Hawthorne wants and not just what Dr Tzakanikis or Mr Hawthorne's family think is best for him (answer 63).

Dr Tzakanikis must make sure that Mr Hawthorne understands the potential benefits and risks of surgery as well as the potential benefits and risks of the principal alternatives to surgery, including the option not to treat (answers 60 and 61).

In itself, Mr Hawthorne's age has no bearing on his ability or otherwise to consent to the referral (answer 62).

64, C; **65**, D; **66**, A; **67**, C

Discussion:

In this scenario, Dr Rauch has to decide whether to press forward with an order to not attempt cardiopulmonary resuscitation (CPR). This decision should be based on clinical factors, not on age – which would be ageism (answer 65).

While it would be good to know Dr Banerjee's motives for requesting a 'do not attempt CPR' order and the opinion of the nursing staff, these shouldn't determine Dr Rauch's decision, which, once again, should be based on clinical factors (answers 64 and 67). Doctors shouldn't make assumptions about a patient's wishes, however frail or elderly the patient may be. Instead, Dr Rauch should sensitively explore Mrs Gosford's willingness and capacity to be involved in a 'do not attempt CPR' decision (answer 66).

68, C; **69**, A; **70**, A; **71**, B

Discussion:

Disclosures in the public interest may be justified when failure to disclose may put the patient or someone else at risk of death or serious harm, or when disclosure is likely to help in the prevention, detection or prosecution of a serious crime (answers 69 and 70).

If practicable, the doctor should seek the patient's consent to the disclosure and tell the patient that a disclosure is being made. However, especially in the case of an anonymous disclosure, the patient's consent isn't essential (answer 71).

A stab wound is a stab wound, regardless of its depth, although this may be one indicator of overall risk (answer 68).

Part IV
The Part of Tens

the part of tens

In this part . . .

✔ Take on board our top ten steps to get you into medical school.

✔ Be sure to check out our top ten ways to manage your stress levels during the application process, and then on through your medical career.

Chapter 13

Ten Steps to Help You Get into Medical or Dental School

*T*he UKCAT is only one part of the overall process of getting into medical or dental school. You need to retain a broader perspective on the challenge you face. In this chapter, we offer some suggestions to help you on the other parts of your journey to medical or dental school.

Deciding Whether Medicine or Dentistry is Right for You

Medicine and dentistry are popular, competitive courses and socially valued professions, but this doesn't mean that one of them is right for you. Make sure that you head down the path of medicine or dentistry because *you* want to, not because other people want you to. To decide whether these fields are for you, try the following:

▶ Work out whether you can see yourself thriving as a doctor or dentist.

▶ Think about the emotional pressure involved in caring for people in pain.

▶ Think about the personal sacrifices it may involve. For example, it may involve temporarily living and working in a part of the country you don't like, especially in the early years. It can sometimes mean postponing having children until you feel more settled in your career, and maybe not seeing as much of your family as you'd like to.

▶ Do some meaningful work experience across a few different settings.

▶ Talk to current students and doctors or dentists.

Achieving the Best Grades

To be successful in your application for medical or dental school, you need to be academically very able. You need excellent GCSEs and a firm expectation of excellent A-levels. Be honest with yourself: if you're not reasonably confident of getting those A-level results, all the work experience – and even the best UKCAT score – in the world won't make a difference.

Doing Your Research

Order – and read – university prospectuses. Go to open days. Read widely about the whole process. Consider attending courses like ours at Get into Medical School (www.getintomedicalschool.org), which explain the medical application process in detail. Know what exams you need to take, when you need to take them, and how to apply for them.

Get Your Personal Statement Right

Start thinking about your UCAS (Universities and Colleges Admission Service) personal statement at an early stage. Identify gaps in your work experience and skills, and plug those gaps before the submission deadline so that your statement is fully rounded. Don't try to do it all at the last minute; personal statements need to be drafted and redrafted many times.

Revising for Your Exams

Both the UKCAT and BMAT exams reward students who've taken the time to familiarise themselves with the tests. This book helps you with the UKCAT, but if you want to apply to a medical school that also requires the BMAT, don't forget to revise for that exam too. Try to get as much practice as possible.

Practising Your Interview Skills

Interviewing is nerve-wracking, especially for first-timers. Make sure that you get plenty of practice in before the big day. Practising interviews with friends is good. Practising interviews with teachers and professionals who are used to interviewing people is better. And practising interviews with people who've already been through medical or dental school interviews is best of all.

Staying Up to Date with Medicine and Dentistry

Medical and dental schools expect candidates to be enthusiastic about medicine and dentistry. You need to have at least a passing familiarity with the world of healthcare and some of the latest news in the field. At www.getintomedicineuk.com, we regularly post healthcare news and highlight some of the key areas for you to consider. Think about setting up a group with any friends who are also applying to medical school, so you can talk further about these areas. See whether any teachers or healthcare professionals are willing to join in with these groups to facilitate the discussion. As well as increasing your familiarity with medicine and dentistry, this will also keep you enthusiastic and motivated.

Sticking to the Timescale

The medical and dental application processes contain a lot of interacting hurdles, many of which have their own submission deadlines and internal administrative annoyances. Use the timeline that we show in Figure 1-1 in Chapter 1 to help you draw up an individualised schedule for your own application.

Reducing Your Anxiety

The application process is long and frustrating. Anxiety is natural but exhausting. Planning ahead, accepting the anxiety as normal, and practising relaxation techniques help reduce your physical and mental agitation. You can find detailed information and more examples in Chapter 14.

Having a Life beyond Medicine or Dentistry

We hope that you get into medical or dental school, but there is a chance that you might not. Regardless of which camp you eventually find yourself in, medicine and dentistry aren't the be-all and end-all of your life. Try hard to retain a sense of personal identity and self-esteem that isn't just tied up with being a doctor or dentist. You'll be a happier and wiser person – and a more effective clinician – if you can manage this.

Chapter 14

Ten Ways to Stay Cool Under Pressure

In This Chapter

▶ Using breathing and relaxation techniques to keep calm

▶ Visualising a positive future

▶ Accepting that some stress is part of the application process

*T*he combination of applying to medical or dental school and sitting exams such as the UKCAT is stressful. Staying calm during the application process is important, however – not only do you feel better, but also you perform better. In this chapter, we suggest ten ways to relax under pressure; you may even find some of these methods are useful in later life if you work as a doctor or dentist.

Keeping Things in Perspective

Becoming a doctor or dentist isn't the be-all and end-all of your life, even if it's very important to you right now. Remember that billions of people live happy, productive, fulfilling lives without working in medicine or dentistry.

Accepting That it's Your Choice

You're voluntarily putting yourself under stress because the potential outcome is something you want to achieve: being a doctor or dentist. You're in control. Acknowledging fundamental truth places the focus of control back in your hands and away from the application system. Your future is yours to decide.

Sticking to Your Plan

You need to be well organised to succeed as a doctor or dentist. Think about when you want to work on your application and exams and when you want to relax.

Draw up a timetable to help you feel in control. Try not to be too fastidious about your plan – it should cover your time in just enough detail to give you a sense of direction without feeling suffocating.

Breathing Deeply

When you feel stressed, your body reacts accordingly, with the so-called *flight or fight reaction*. Your pulse quickens, your muscles tense up, and your breathing becomes faster and shallower. The good news is that the relationship is two way: if you can notice these changes and act to control them, you can make yourself feel calmer. By consciously slowing down your breathing and making each breath deeper and more controlled, you can calm and focus your thoughts.

Try breathing in deeply through your nose and then breathing out slowly through slightly pursed lips, taking about five seconds to complete an entire cycle. You don't need to actively time your breathing – just breathe a little more slowly than normal, but not so slowly that you feel uncomfortable.

The first time you try this, you'll probably lose concentration after a few breaths, but if you keep practising you'll get better at the technique. Eventually, the technique becomes second nature when you're stressed, and can really work wonders in relaxing your mind and body.

Relaxing Progressively

Consciously relaxing your muscles reduces the tension that builds up with prolonged stress. Practise alternately tensing and relaxing your muscles under conscious control. To do this, follow these steps:

1. **Start off by scrunching up your feet, holding them tensed for a few seconds, and then letting them gradually relax over another few seconds.**

2. **Repeat Step 1 with your feet a few times and move on to your calf muscles, your thighs, your fists, arms, and so on, all the way up to your forehead muscles.**

   The whole sequence can take some minutes, but think of it as a break from working and worrying.

Like deep controlled breathing, your muscle relaxation technique will improve with practice, so keep trying.

Trying Visualisation Exercises

You can use visualisation techniques to help you relax and to build your confidence.

To use visualisation for relaxation, follow these steps:

1. **Sit or lie down for a few moments.**

2. **Close your eyes and think of a time and a place where you were very happy.**

   Try to recall all the physical, sensory and emotional details of the event. Relive the event as closely as you can.

3. **Rest within the moment.**

   You can supplement the visualisation with the deep breathing technique to boost its relaxing effect.

4. **When you feel rested, slowly open your eyes, let yourself become aware of your surroundings again and take another deep breath before returning to work.**

To build your confidence with visualisation, focus on the successful outcome. Imagine yourself in the position of passing your exams with flying colours, getting into medical or dental school, and qualifying as a doctor or dentist. If it feels like tempting fate, challenge your fear of failure instead of leaving it to fester in your subconscious mind. Aim for success and give yourself permission to see yourself as a successful person. Many of the world's top sportspeople use visualisation techniques to help them focus before major competitions.

Becoming Familiar with the Application Process

The unknown is a terrifying empty space. You project your deepest and darkest fears into that empty space. If you haven't practised enough UKCAT questions or revised for your A-levels, your fear of the unknown can overwhelm you. By familiarising yourself with all the elements of the medical or dental school application process, you get comfortable with the steps you need to take. Familiarity acts as a reassuring protective shield around you. If you haven't researched the application process much, Part I and Chapter 13 of this book are good places to start.

Steering Clear of Denial

Stress and anxiety are a normal part of life – and of university applications. Many of the other tips in this chapter can help you control your stress and anxiety. However stressful you find the process of applying to medical or dental school, don't try to run away or use alcohol or drugs to block things out – denial never works in the long term and can lead to more problems and distress.

Avoiding Upsetting Other People

When you feel stressed, you may take out your pent-up frustration on other people – usually those closest to you. Your friends and family love you, so we hope they forgive you to some extent if you don't act like yourself when under the stress of applying to medical or dental school. But instead of upsetting people, try to use some of the stress-busting techniques included in this chapter. After all, distressing your family and friends only adds to your stress.

Taking a Break

Remember that the application process is a marathon not a sprint. If you work at 100 per cent effort throughout the process, you'll burn yourself out. Take time out to do the things you love and be with the people you like. By unwinding and relaxing, you'll be much more effective when you go back to work.

Index

• *V* •

• *W* •

Notes

Notes

Notes

Notes

Notes

Notes

Notes

About the Authors

Dr Chris Chopdar MA(Oxon), BMBCh (Oxon), MRCPsych is co-founder of Get into Medical School Ltd, which has a strong track record of getting prospective medical students into the university of their choice. He enjoys teaching courses both in Oxford and at schools and colleges across the UK. Chris got his medical degree from Oxford University, and also has a Master's degree in Physiological Sciences from his time there.

He returned to Oxford as a psychiatrist after brief stints working in other parts of the country. Chris continues in clinical practice, combining this work with interests in interview technique and the psychological motifs inherent in clothing.

Dr Neel Burton BSc, MBBS, MRCPsych, MA(Phil), AKC is co-founder of Get into Medical School Ltd. He designed its UKCAT course and also coaches individual UKCAT candidates.

He qualified in medicine from the University of London and is now a psychiatrist, philosopher and writer. He is the recipient of Society of Authors Richard Asher Prize, the British Medical Association's Young Authors' Award, and the Medical Journalists' Association Open Book Award. He is happy to talk at charities, schools, universities, and other public gatherings.

Dedication

We would like to dedicate this book to the many students we've taught over the years. Their intellectual curiosity makes teaching a pleasure, and through the teaching, we ourselves continue to learn.

Authors' Acknowledgments

The Roman philosopher and statesman Seneca once said, 'A gift consists not in what is done or given, but in the intention of the giver or doer'. Your authors have been fortunate indeed in the intentions of those around them.

Chris would particularly like to thank his father for his ongoing encouragement and support, and his late mother for instilling in him a sense of curiosity about the world.

Chris and Neel extend their joint gratitude to the entire *For Dummies* team at Wiley. Creating this second edition was in some respects a more complicated process than the first edition. The UKCAT exam changed significantly and we wanted to expand the text and questions to reflect that change. Doing that while keeping the book accessible and useful was challenging, and we're grateful to everyone at Wiley for their support during this process. Special thanks go to commissioning editor Mike Baker and development editors Jo Jones (first edition) and Simon Bell (second edition) for their shared ability to balance attention to detail with overall vision. Thanks also to the illustrators, who must have sometimes felt like pulling their hair out with frustration when faced with the task of neatly reproducing the complicated diagrams used in the practice tests. Finally, we must acknowledge the patience and diligence of our copy and technical editors. We certainly appreciate their efforts, and are confident that so will all those students who successfully use this book to prepare for the UKCAT.

Publisher's Acknowledgments

We're proud of this book; please send us your comments at http://dummies.custhelp.com. For other comments, please contact our Customer Care Department within the U.S. at 877-762-2974, outside the U.S. at (001) 317-572-3993, or fax 317-572-4002.

Some of the people who helped bring this book to market include the following:

Acquisitions, Editorial, and Vertical Websites

Project Editor: Simon Bell

   (Previous Edition: Jo Jones)

Commissioning Editor: Mike Baker

Assistant Editor: Ben Kemble

Development Editor: Simon Bell

Copy Editor: Mary White

Technical Editors: Sam Harrison, Amy Nicklin, Alix Godfrey

Proofreader: Kim Vernon

Production Manager: Daniel Mersey

Publisher: Miles Kendall

Vertical Websites: Rich Graves

Cover Photos: ©uchar/iStockphoto.com

Project Coordinator: Melissa Cossell

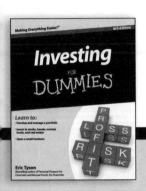
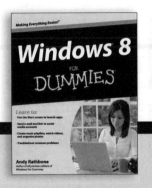
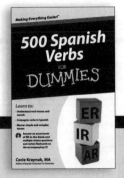
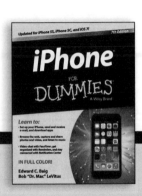

Math & Science

Algebra I For Dummies,
2nd Edition
978-0-470-55964-2

Anatomy and Physiology
For Dummies, 2nd Edition
978-0-470-92326-9

Astronomy For Dummies,
3rd Edition
978-1-118-37697-3

Biology For Dummies,
2nd Edition
978-0-470-59875-7

Chemistry For Dummies,
2nd Edition
978-1-118-00730-3

1001 Algebra II Practice
Problems For Dummies
978-1-118-44662-1

Microsoft Office

Excel 2013 For Dummies
978-1-118-51012-4

Office 2013 All-in-One
For Dummies
978-1-118-51636-2

PowerPoint 2013
For Dummies
978-1-118-50253-2

Word 2013 For Dummies
978-1-118-49123-2

Music

Blues Harmonica
For Dummies
978-1-118-25269-7

Guitar For Dummies,
3rd Edition
978-1-118-11554-1

iPod & iTunes
For Dummies, 10th Edition
978-1-118-50864-0

Programming

Beginning Programming
with C For Dummies
978-1-118-73763-7

Excel VBA Programming
For Dummies, 3rd Edition
978-1-118-49037-2

Java For Dummies,
6th Edition
978-1-118-40780-6

Religion & Inspiration

The Bible For Dummies
978-0-7645-5296-0

Buddhism For Dummies,
2nd Edition
978-1-118-02379-2

Catholicism For Dummies,
2nd Edition
978-1-118-07778-8

Self-Help & Relationships

Beating Sugar Addiction
For Dummies
978-1-118-54645-1

Meditation For Dummies,
3rd Edition
978-1-118-29144-3

Seniors

Laptops For Seniors
For Dummies, 3rd Edition
978-1-118-71105-7

Computers For Seniors
For Dummies, 3rd Edition
978-1-118-11553-4

iPad For Seniors
For Dummies, 6th Edition
978-1-118-72826-0

Social Security
For Dummies
978-1-118-20573-0

Smartphones & Tablets

Android Phones
For Dummies, 2nd Edition
978-1-118-72030-1

Nexus Tablets
For Dummies
978-1-118-77243-0

Samsung Galaxy S 4
For Dummies
978-1-118-64222-1

Samsung Galaxy Tabs
For Dummies
978-1-118-77294-2

Test Prep

ACT For Dummies,
5th Edition
978-1-118-01259-8

ASVAB For Dummies,
3rd Edition
978-0-470-63760-9

GRE For Dummies,
7th Edition
978-0-470-88921-3

Officer Candidate Tes
For Dummies
978-0-470-59876-4

Physician's Assistant
For Dummies
978-1-118-11556-5

Series 7 Exam For Du
978-0-470-09932-2

Windows 8

Windows 8.1 All-in-O
For Dummies
978-1-118-82087-2

Windows 8.1 For Dun
978-1-118-82121-3

Windows 8.1 For Dun
Book + DVD Bundle
978-1-118-82107-7

ℯ Available in print and e-book formats.

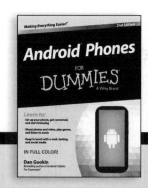
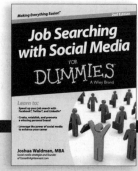
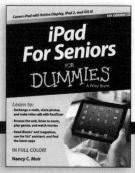
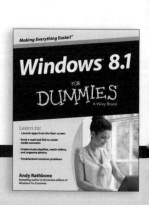

Available wherever books are sold. **For more information or to order direct visit www.dummies.com**

Take Dummies with you everywhere you go!

Whether you are excited about e-books, want more from the web, must have your mobile apps, or are swept up in social media, Dummies makes everything easier.

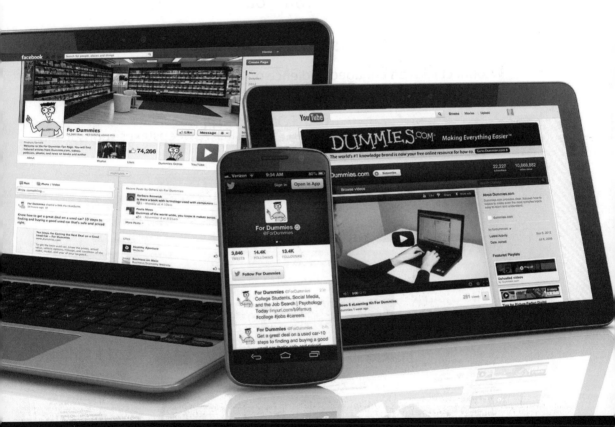

For Dummies is the global leader in the reference category and one of the most trusted and highly regarded brands in the world. No longer just focused on books, customers now have access to the For Dummies content they need in the format they want. Let us help you develop a solution that will fit your brand and help you connect with your customers.

Advertising & Sponsorships

Connect with an engaged audience on a powerful multimedia site, and position your message alongside expert how-to content.

Targeted ads • Video • Email marketing • Microsites • Sweepstakes sponsorship

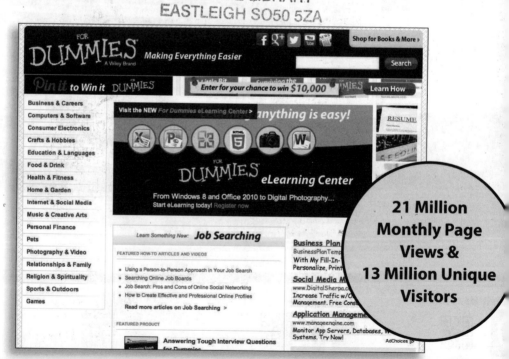